NATURAL THERAPIES

Edited by

MARGOT MCCARTHY

Thorsons
An Imprint of HarperCollins*Publishers*

Thorsons
An Imprint of HarperCollins*Publishers*
77–85 Fulham Palace Road,
Hammersmith, London W6 8JB
1160 Battery Street,
San Francisco, California 94111–1213

Published by Thorsons 1994
1   3   5   7   9   10   8   6   4   2

A catalogue record for this book
is available from the British Library

ISBN 0 7225 2830 2

Typeset by Harper Phototypesetters Limited
Northampton, England
Printed in Great Britain by
Mackays of Chatham plc, Chatham, Kent

To my father, Jim Gilchrist

✑ CONTENTS ✑

❧ ACKNOWLEDGEMENTS ❧

I would like to express my thanks to the therapists at Neal's Yard Therapy Rooms for their contributions to this book, to the editorial staff at Thorsons who have provided so much support throughout, and finally to my husband, Keith, whose help and encouragement has made this book a reality.

PART ONE

ALTERNATIVE MEDICINE

❧ An Overview ❧

What Is Alternative/Complementary Medicine?

It has become increasingly clear, both to the medical establishment and the general public, that alternative forms of medicine make a positive and successful contribution to health care today. It has become obvious that no one system of medicine has the complete answer to all our health care requirements. Each system has a place and application. We should be aware of the value and efficacy of the various types of treatment, be they orthodox or those that we have come to call 'alternative' or 'complementary'.

The term 'alternative' is in itself confusing for it is used to cover many diverse approaches to healing, some of which appear unorthodox even to practitioners of 'conventional alternative' therapies. At Neal's Yard Therapy Rooms we concentrate on the mainstream alternative therapies. The treatments we offer fall basically into three groups: structural therapies, vital-force therapies and psychotherapies. This is of course an over-simplification, for therapies frequently merge more than one of these methodologies toward a more precise and balanced approach, but it does help in an understanding of the different starting points.

The structural therapies – Chiropractic and Osteopathy, for example – deal in the physical manipulation of the body parts, to rectify physical injury or maladjustment.

The vital-force type therapies take a more subtle approach and probe deeper into the whole symptom/lifestyle picture. The treatments employed by this group are often aimed at stimulation of our own built-in healing processes.

The Psychotherapies – for example Psychotherapy, Counselling or Hypnotherapy – approach healing from a more cerebral direction.

WHO CAN BENEFIT?

Despite ever-increasing costs, the availability of modern drugs and sophisticated surgical techniques, conventional medicine treats more people each year, many of these on the treadmill of ongoing treatment. Many diseases remain a mystery with no known cure, and new diseases become prevalent with no known cause. Established medical practice is failing to understand the root cause of ill health. This approach to healing concentrates on the alleviation of specific symptoms, sometimes with techniques that conceal problems rather than cure them or that cause the imbalance to manifest itself in other symptoms. Clearly conventional medicine is failing to restore people to harmony and balanced health.

The validity of any healing treatment can only be judged by the complete return to well-being of the individual. The problem arises in matching, to each patient, the most appropriate treatment, to ensure the return to well-being in the safest, most complete way possible. During the last 20 years we have seen an enormous increase in the awareness that there are and have been for centuries, systems of healing other than the conventional 20th-century type, which offer a more complete and natural approach to our health needs. Many people are now taking the initiative for themselves and questioning conventional medical thinking and rightfully concluding that it is not always the best path. Patients have become increasingly disillusioned, causing them to seek out more complete health care systems. These systems are what we offer, not to replace conventional medicine but to supplement it, giving the opportunity for a more natural complete healing.

The orthodox approach to disease is based on the consideration of a given set of symptoms presented by a patient, taking little or no account of the deeper problems that caused the manifestation of these symptoms. If these symptoms are relieved, the patient is considered cured. But can it be that simple? Disease can often be the outward manifestation of inner disharmony, the symptoms a signpost to a deeper imbalance. The alleviation of unpleasant, often painful symptoms is of course an objective – but how much more satisfactory both to relieve the symptoms and to reach the root cause of the problem. Alternative medicine tries to provide a framework for people to explore the cause of disease and to consider the deeper hidden problem.

WHAT IS SELF-HEALING?

Every person has the potential of self-healing. Consider the placebo, a healing effect from an ineffectual substance. This effect is often dismissed and we frequently hear it said that the success of a substance or approach was 'merely' placebo. But surely this effect shows something of vital importance. The healing clearly does not come from the placebo but from the mind, which is inspired to heal for itself, using resources that are already at its disposal. The mind miraculously corrects the imbalance for itself. This is undeniable: the systems for healing already exist within each of us. The role of some therapists is therefore that of a catalyst: theirs is the ability to tap into, mobilize and support these inner resources; to cause the whole to unite against the offending symptoms; to restore the true balance.

Health should be a personal responsibility. We have been encouraged into passivity, expecting 'someone else' to right the problem – our problem. Disease should be seen within the context of an entire life: it forces people to appraise their complete lifestyle;

it can be a signal for change. The correct advice can actually lead to better health and a more harmonious existence.

❧ Choosing the Right Therapy❧

Selecting a Therapy

Matching a patient's complaint to a suitable therapy can be self-evident, but occasionally this is problematic. Sometimes more than one therapy is employed during a course of treatment. A number of therapies may, on the surface, seem appropriate for a particular condition, but only one will be outstanding when considering a particular individual. People's response to therapy is varied, because as individuals we have different tolerance levels/response times, etc. Some therapies work well in conjunction with others, while other combinations should be avoided. Used simultaneously, certain major therapies – for example, Homoeopathy and Aromatherapy – confuse the patient's response and can make it difficult to evaluate any reactions effectively. The strong volatile nature of the essential oils used in Aromatherapy will negate the effect of subtle Homoeopathic remedies, for example. It is strongly advised not to mix and match therapies without professional guidance.

The reception area of any clinic is frequently a public space, with telephones ringing, patients making bookings and others awaiting appointments. This is certainly not the ideal place for prospective clients to outline their personal problems. For this reason advisory sessions should be available in an area separate from reception, where patients feel comfortable and relaxed. During this session, prospective patients are encouraged to expand on the nature of their problem, enabling a therapist to reach a considered judgement and give guidance while, at the same time, allowing the prospective patient to reach a decision without feeling pressured.

An advisory session should address itself to three main points:

1. Ascertaining the main problem, be it mental, physical or emotional.
2. Looking at the patient as a 'whole' and not fragmenting the patient's complaint from other areas of his or her life.
3. Selecting the optimum treatment available for that particular individual, not just for the complaint.

The importance of discussing a problem and the desired outcome can be illustrated by looking at a client presenting severe symptoms of stress. Stress can be approached from several directions using different therapies, according to the symptoms shown, the personality of the client and the outcome sought. Stress has varied manifestations: physical, emotional or mental or a combination of the three. The first thing to point out is that while stress frequently plays a negative role in our lives, it cannot be eradicated; it is our *attitude* to stress and learning to recognize, adjust and cope with it in a more positive way that count. If anxiety and insomnia are the symptoms presented, then help can be offered with a physically relaxing type of therapy such as Massage, Aromatherapy or Shiatsu.

A frequent response to stress is the subconscious tightening of muscles; an inability to relax these muscles leads to chronic muscular tension which in turn can lead to migraines, headaches, etc. To alleviate and break down this physical tension a physically relaxing therapy may be suggested: Aromatherapy, Yoga, Shiatsu, deep-tissue massage or Rolfing. Ongoing activities such as Yoga or the Alexander Technique can help maintain a more relaxed state.

Mental and emotional stress may require Hypnotherapy, Psychotherapy or Counselling. Some clients would prefer a more enquiring approach in dealing with stress, in as much as they want to be able to control it and minimize its effect, in which case Neuro-Linguistic Programming (NLP) or Autogenic Training might be suggested. As can be seen, the therapy chosen must be considered individually for each client, taking into account his or her desires and expectations as well as the obvious elimination of basic symptoms.

Patients frequently opt for a therapy that has proved effective for a friend, colleague or family member. If this therapy proves appropriate to their condition, it is helpful, as they already have a degree of confidence in its efficacy. Some have a particular interest in or some degree of knowledge of a particular therapy, which naturally gives them some confidence in that form of treatment. Others are drawn inexplicably towards one type of treatment without apparent reason. If the intuitive feeling is strong it is as well to trust it. Such people are likely to be open to this treatment at this particular time in their lives and will respond well to it.

Health is a personal responsibility. The selection of a therapy is entirely up to you. The role of the adviser is not to coerce potential patients into one type of therapy as opposed to another, but to ensure that they make an informed choice and that they feel comfortable with their decision. You should never be pushed into making a decision; if you require time to contemplate, so much the better, as the choice reached will be from your own endeavour and you will have played an active part in your own personal health plan. Time taken to read and find out more about the different therapies is extremely worthwhile, increasing your understanding of the form the treatment will take.

It is important to bear in mind that the treatment itself should not be stressful; it should fit comfortably into your daily routine. If visiting a complementary medicine clinic involves a lengthy journey or difficulties with domestic arrangements it may be suggested that you see a practitioner closer to home. You can be given addresses and details of self-help groups, networks and other sources of assistance as is appropriate. It is important to create an awareness of methods of self-help outside of the treatment sessions, as this can enhance the benefits you get from a therapy.

WHAT HAPPENS ON A FIRST VISIT FOR TREATMENT?

First visits vary considerably depending on the particular therapy chosen. However, many share certain features. For most therapies the first appointment is longer than subsequent ones because, having taken the case history, treatment is then given. Subsequent visits are shorter as they consist purely of an update from you and further treatment. The therapist will discuss how many visits he or she feels will be required to clear the current problem and what the prognosis is. Sometimes referral to another therapist may be suggested, as would be the case if when seeing a Homoeopath for the treatment of headaches, an old whiplash injury is mentioned. The Homoeopath might then refer you to an Osteopath or Chiropractor to check there is no spinal displacement present before proceeding with treatment.

Initially a therapist will be interested in the symptoms of your current complaint. You will be asked the usual personal details, such as your age, occupation and so on. Details of your present condition will be noted and discussed at length – how and when it began and the course it has followed. Past medical history, both personal and that of your family is relevant, as many problems are deeply rooted. Questions relating to diet, sleep patterns and your general lifestyle are common to build up a picture of the overall person. Frequently additional information may be required, regarding relationships, habits and behavioural patterns. Detailed information enables the therapist to reach an understanding of the underlying problem that has caused your symptoms to occur, and to make an early diagnosis. Many therapists also make a routine physical examination, recording your pulse and blood pressure, etc.

Some therapies use particular diagnostic methods: for example, Herbalists and Acupuncturists make a tongue diagnosis, as the state of health can be reflected in the colour, texture and coatings of the tongue. Pulse points (not the same as for an orthodox pulse reading) may be palpated to ascertain energy flow and rhythms.

When seeing an Osteopath or Chiropractor it may be suggested that you have an X-ray, in which case the therapist will organize this for you. If you are already in possession of X-rays it would be advisable to bring these along with you.

What to Expect/Look for/Check-Up On

People, generally, have only limited experience of health care, perhaps only ever having consulted a GP or made a visit to a local hospital. Thus a first visit to an Alternative Health Clinic can be stressful. People, when ill, are especially sensitive and vulnerable, many are in pain and so it is extremely important for a clinic to allay the tension and anxiety that are naturally felt. It is essential that receptionists are sensitive and patient, ready to answer all your queries and deal professionally with your needs. The atmosphere should be relaxed but efficient. The qualifications and details of the practising therapists should be readily available in the reception area and the receptionist competent to offer practical advice.

First impressions are always important. Establish the range of available therapies, assess how you are received and informed and the feeling of the environment. Information should always be available on the variety of treatments offered and, better still, on complementary activities – for example, local classes, activities, group meetings, talks, lectures, etc.

Before deciding upon a specific course of therapy it may be appropriate to talk to a couple of therapists of different disciplines to ascertain which particular therapy may be the most appropriate. Receptionists can usually organize these informal chats with the therapists available. Many therapies interact with others quite satisfactorily, but it should be noted that it is best not to mix two major therapies for the same problem. Always check with the relevant therapists if you are contemplating combining any forms of treatment.

Fees

Regarding fees, it is often difficult to know what is the 'right' price for treatments. It has to be remembered that high overheads and running costs face all central London clinics; fees at any city clinic will be higher than in rural areas or for therapists who practise from their homes. A price list should be available so that you understand the financial commitment you are undertaking. In many instances, a first appointment is longer since a detailed case history has to be taken, with subsequent visits being shorter. For example, a first appointment with a Homoeopath can take up to 1½ hours, while subsequent visits will be 30 to 45 minutes. Fees, therefore, may be higher for the first visit and lower subsequently. You should also determine whether the fees include any herbal or Homoeopathic prescription or if this would be extra. Many clients have private health insurance; the costs of treatment can be met in this way. Patients should inform their health insurance company of the therapist concerned and, if appropriate, cover will be given.

Qualifications

Entrusting your health to somebody else can be an extremely worrying idea. Are the therapists qualified? What do their qualifications actually mean? Do they know what they are doing? Will they take adequate care of you? Will they advise you as to what is best for your condition? These are all very common and realistic concerns. Because of the current state of affairs in the UK, there is no specific legislation in place to monitor the training or qualification of therapists. In order to check a therapist's qualifications you need to be able to recognize a *bona fide* qualification. This is unfortunately easier said than done, with the variety of training establishments that abound in Britain today. Some courses available are weekend or correspondence courses, with no practical training involved. It should be recognized that many of these courses merely offer a taster to various subjects and that proper training is a far more lengthy and involved regime.

The authorizing bodies of the various therapies produce membership lists and directories of qualified practitioners. Membership of these bodies is restricted to practitioners who have undergone training at a recognized establishment where stringent professional criteria have been met, to ensure high standards and conformity to a code of ethics.

Anxious patients should be assured that if the training course undertaken has been approved by the relevant Register/Society this ensures standards of training and competence. The Institute for Complementary Medicine is a body which checks the credentials of training establishments and can offer advice and comment on the types of training offered. Also there is the British Register of Complementary Practitioners, which provides national listings of qualified practitioners in the major disciplines.

British Complementary Medicine Association
Mental Health Unit
St Charles' Hospital
Exmoor Street
London W10 6DZ
Tel. 081–964 1205

British Holistic Medical Association
179 Gloucester Place
London NW1 6DX
Tel. 071–262 5299

British Register of Complementary Practitioners
Institute of Complementary Medicine
PO Box 194
London SE16 1QZ
Tel. 071–237 5165

The Council for Complementary and Alternative Medicine
179 Gloucester Place
London NW1 6DX
Tel. 071–724 9103

Natural Health Network (Association of Alternative Health
Centres & Practitioners)
Chardstock House
Chard
Somerset TA20 2TL
Tel. 0460 63229

Theosophical Society of England
50 Gloucester Place
London W1H 3HJ
Tel. 071–935 9261

Australia
Australasian College of Natural Therapies
620 Harris Street
Ultimo NSW 2007
Tel. 02 212 6699

Australian Natural Therapists Association Ltd
PO Box 522
Sutherland NSW 2232
Tel. 02 521 2063

A QUICK GUIDE TO FINDING THE RIGHT THERAPY AND PRACTITIONER

1. Decide on which therapy you think will be right for you.
2. Find a therapist from an established clinic/centre/professional register.
3. Inform your own GP if you are already undergoing orthodox treatment for your complaint.

What to Ask

1. Can the practitioner help with treatment for your particular complaint?
2. Has the therapist previous experience of treating this condition?
3. How much does treatment cost, and how long is each treatment session?
4. What is the plan of actual treatment, the likely responses, how long it might take, the prognosis.

What to Check

1. The therapist's credentials: training, qualifications, membership of appropriate professional body (which should include: code of ethics, public register, disciplinary procedures and complaints mechanism and insurance).
2. Professional attitude of the therapist, other practitioners and staff at the clinic.
3. Standards of hygiene.
4. Quality of advice and how much time given to you by staff at the clinic and by the practitioner.
5. Do you fit in? – empathy with people and place. Do you feel at ease and comfortable?

NEAL'S YARD THERAPY ROOMS

In the early 1970s the long-established fruit and vegetable market at London's Covent Garden was transferred to a more practical site at Nine Elms; consequently a great number of old warehouses and stables were left vacant, many of them in a semi-derelict state. Considering the central location occupied by these premises there was exciting potential for radical change. Opportunities for new businesses abounded and the whole structure and atmosphere of the Garden was to change.

Nicholas Saunders was one individual who recognized the potential to implement and develop many of his somewhat unorthodox ideas of retailing and business. With great enthusiasm and purpose he set about implementing his schemes and within a short period he had opened the Neal's Yard Warehouse which retailed wholefoods in bulk quantities. There followed Neal's Yard Dairy, specializing in British cheeses; the Monmouth Street Coffee House; Neal's Yard Bakery (run on co-operative ideals); Neal's Yard Apothecary; and Neal's Yard Soup and Salad Bar, all within a relatively short time.

Saunders then turned his attention to alternative health, the outcome of a long-standing interest in the subject. He opened six therapy rooms on the second floor of No. 2 Neal's Yard, an old warehouse, and offered these as practising space to a variety of trained alternative health therapists.

Thus Neal's Yard Therapy Rooms commenced in the summer of 1982. With the ever-burgeoning public interest and awareness that alternative health could offer an effective option to orthodox medical treatment, more therapists were encouraged to start practices. I [Margot McCarthy] became involved with the Therapy Rooms in the Spring of 1983, while training as a Homoeopath. Gradually more and more rooms were let and the opening hours extended to fulfil growing client demand. In spite of operating in such a confined area – some 450 sq ft/42 sq m – we managed to see some 10,000 patients annually. In 1991, the first floor of the building became available and it was decided that there was room for expansion; subsequently another four treatment rooms were added, with a more spacious reception area overlooking the yard below. We now see some 15,000 patients annually and have been able to broaden the range of therapies available.

Many therapists apply to practise at Neal's Yard; their selection is always carefully monitored to ensure the maintenance of high standards of treatment and care, a reputation of which we are justifiably proud.

New legislation has made it permissible for GPs to utilize the services of alternative practitioners within their practices, which ultimately provides patients with a more rounded and balanced health care system, allowing greater scope for holistic treatment. With changing attitudes within the orthodox medical system, we benefit from referrals from GPs who now realize that alternative therapies are sometimes more appropriate to their patients' needs than standard orthodox treatment. Alternative and orthodox medicine can run in tandem; there is a place within any health care system for both forms of treatment, whichever happens to be appropriate to the individual. The main factor has to be that, in considering the options available, the patient can make a personal choice as to which type of treatment will suit, which feels most comfortable. Ultimately the fact that the patient is able to take responsibility for and play an active role in his or her own health care is paramount.

Many clients come to Neal's Yard Therapy Rooms after a long period of orthodox treatment. Some, having experienced many hospital outpatient appointments, having been seen by varying ranks of doctors and having had to explain their problem many times, are naturally wary. At Neal's Yard we try to ensure that patients are relaxed; we provide continuity of care (a patient will see the same practitioner at each visit and not be passed from pillar to post). Being ill is stressful enough; patients should not feel even more stressed by mishandled appointments, staff who show little concern or unprofessional therapists. Unlike at NHS hospitals and clinics here in Britain, our staff do not wear uniforms and steer away from the rather cold clinical atmosphere that all too frequently reminds patients of lengthy and trying hospital visits.

At Neal's Yard we also provide a 'Therapists Book' to prospective patients. All therapists have to submit a clear CV stating details of training, dates and qualifications gained, membership of professional organizations, post-graduate experience, the manner in which they work, fees and length of appointment times, so that patients have the relevant information presented to them in a clear and direct manner. To train as a therapist requires considerable time and effort. A therapist needs to demonstrate a high level of commitment and competence in order to qualify. All therapists who practise at Neal's Yard are professionally registered and insured, thus protecting patients' interests.

With thousands of people now working in the Covent Garden area we have a wide catchment area which yields a very cosmopolitan clientele. Many patients appreciate the fact that we remain open until 9.30 p.m. daily, so that they can benefit from treatment after working hours. Most of our 60 therapists practise on two or three days per week; the rest of their time is taken up by practices at home or in other clinics, or by teaching commitments. Having such a central location makes it easy for patients to visit from all areas of London and even further afield.

Our clients come from all walks of life, from the very young to the elderly, and from a wide variety of professions. Alternative health is applicable to everybody. Neal's Yard also acts as an information point: we are frequently asked for addresses of centres and practitioners from as far afield as Warsaw and Wellington, New Zealand. Over the years we have been able to accrue a great deal of information relating to the many different types of therapies available, and keep many of the registers of trained therapists so that we are able to offer advice to the public whether they happen to be in London or not.

We maintain close links with the other related businesses in the Yard, especially Neal's Yard Remedies and East–West Herbs. Many of our patients are able to obtain their Herbal or Homoeopathic prescriptions at these outlets, and many who seek self-help for a chronic condition are frequently advised to see a professional therapist and are thus referred to us.

People who come to Neal's Yard Therapy Rooms seeking advice and help are beginning to accept responsibility for their own health. It is our duty to ensure that they have all the options put clearly before them to encourage this new-found responsibility.

PART TWO

BODY SYSTEMS

∾ INTRODUCTION∾

The following sections describing the various systems of the body are aimed at the lay reader who may have only a vague knowledge, or have forgotten since schooldays how the body functions. This is only a very simplified overview of each system, with many finer details of function omitted. There are many fine textbooks concerned with anatomy and physiology describing each system more fully if you wish to pursue study in any area. It is hoped that through these sections you may be able to grasp a basic idea of the way the body actually works and will come to understand how all the systems are inextricably linked.

CARDIOVASCULAR SYSTEM

Everything needed to sustain life is carried within the bloodstream. The heart is the blood's 'central pumping station'.

The Heart

The heart is a hollow muscular organ and lies between the lungs in the *thoracic cavity*. There are three layers: the endocardium (the lining), the myocardium (the strong cardiac muscle, which makes up the greater part of the heart) and the pericardium (the double outer covering which contains pericardial fluid preventing friction as the heart moves).

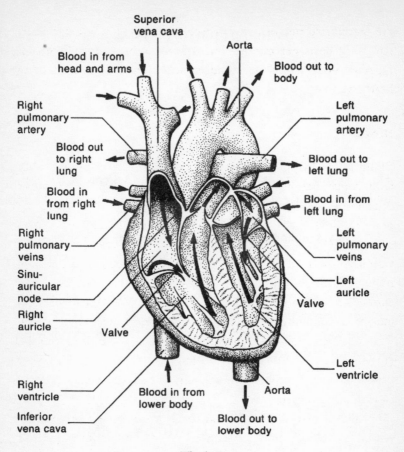

Superior vena cava

Blood in from head and arms

Aorta

Blood out to body

Right pulmonary artery

Left pulmonary artery

Blood out to right lung

Blood out to left lung

Blood in from right lung

Blood in from left lung

Right pulmonary veins

Left pulmonary veins

Sinu-auricular node

Left auricle

Right auricle

Valve

Valve

Left ventricle

Right ventricle

Blood in from lower body

Aorta

Inferior vena cava

Blood out to lower body

The heart

The heart is basically two pumps: one responsible for sending oxygenated blood around the body and the other for returning deoxygenated blood to the lungs to be reoxygenated. The two 'sides' of the heart are entirely separate from one another. Each side is comprised of two interconnecting chambers (atrium and ventricle). The left side has the harder task, pumping freshly oxygenated blood out into the arteries to be circulated around the body. The right side pumps deoxygenated blood the short distance to the lungs for reoxygenation.

The heart muscle contracts automatically, the rate controlled by the autonomic nervous system (see page 35). The average heart rate is 72 beats per minute, but this varies between individuals. Exercise, body temperature and emotional state all influence the heart rate.

Blood

Blood is the major transportation system of the body. An adult body contains about $5^1/9$ pints, carried through thousands of miles of blood vessels. Blood is composed of a variety of constituents, 55 per cent of the total blood volume being plasma, the straw-coloured medium in which red and white blood cells, platelets and various essential chemicals are found. White blood cells are mainly responsible for protecting the body against disease, by producing antibodies in response to disease agents for both instant use and long-term immunity. Red blood cells transport the oxygen in the form of haemoglobin. Platelets are responsible for maintaining the correct blood-clotting times, too few resulting in a tendency to bruise and bleed easily, too many resulting in a tendency to form clots in inappropriate places.

A balance of healthy cells has to be maintained continuously within the blood. The destruction of old cells via the liver and spleen and the production of new ones from the bone marrow perpetuate this delicate balance.

Blood has two functions: transportation and protection.

TRANSPORTATION
Nutrients from the digestive system are passed to all cells of the body by the blood, as is oxygen collected from the lungs. Waste materials are collected from the cells and carried away to be excreted. Hormones from the endocrine system are distributed, antibodies are taken to sites of infection and heat is carried from active areas to less active ones and to the skin for dispersal.

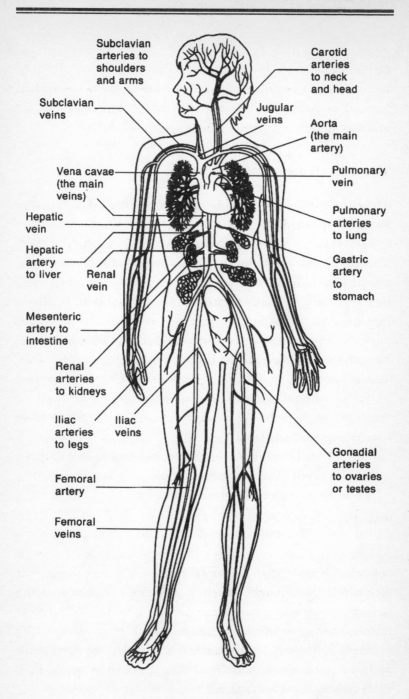

Subclavian arteries to shoulders and arms

Carotid arteries to neck and head

Subclavian veins

Jugular veins

Aorta (the main artery)

Vena cavae (the main veins)

Pulmonary vein

Hepatic vein

Pulmonary arteries to lung

Hepatic artery to liver

Gastric artery to stomach

Renal vein

Mesenteric artery to intestine

Renal arteries to kidneys

Iliac arteries to legs

Iliac veins

Femoral artery

Gonadial arteries to ovaries or testes

Femoral veins

The circulatory system

PROTECTION

Protection of the system is maintained by clotting, to exclude harmful organisms and prevent blood loss. White cells combat invading organisms and help in healing wounds.

The Circulatory Network

The circulatory network can be seen with the heart at its centre. Freshly oxygenated blood from the lungs flows into the left side of the heart via the pulmonary vein and is pumped into the aorta. This then feeds the entire body through a series of branching arteries which divide into smaller arterioles; they in turn divide into a network of tiny capillaries, through whose walls the blood supplies oxygen and nutrients to the cells and collects the waste products. The capillaries merge into venules and then into veins to carry the deoxygenated blood back to the right side of the heart. The heart then pumps the deoxygenated blood into the pulmonary artery to the lungs for reoxygenation.

As blood is pumped around the body under pressure, arteries have thicker, stronger walls than veins. As most blood pressure is dissipated before entering a vein, the return to the heart is aided by a series of valves contained within the veins.

The Lymph System

The lymph system is the body's secondary circulatory system. It comprises lymph glands, in some instances grouped together to form nodes, and lymph vessels. There is no central pumping station for this system; muscular activity is responsible for the movement of this fluid around the body.

Lymph is similar to blood plasma; it acts to bathe the cells of the body and collect up plasma which has escaped into the tissues from the bloodstream at capillary level.

Scattered throughout the lymph drainage system are glands

which are able to produce the special disease-fighting cells called lymphocytes and plasma cells. Some of these disease-fighting cells do not remain within the lymph glands but are shed into the lymph drainage system. If their production is stepped up because of infection, these glands can become hard and tender or painful to the touch.

There is also lymph tissue found in the adenoids, tonsils, parts of the intestine, spleen and, in children, in the thymus (which later shrivels).

THE SPLEEN

The spleen is found beneath the diaphragm and to the left and behind the stomach. It is responsible for the quality control of the blood in circulation, by acting as a reservoir for all kinds of blood cells and by breaking down worn-out red blood cells. It is also responsible for producing new red blood cells in the foetus (and occasionally in the adult after severe blood loss). It also produces lymphocytes from the lymph tissue within it.

RESPIRATORY SYSTEM

Respiration

Respiration is the process that fulfils our body's need for oxygen and the removal of waste gases. This is achieved through a three-part sequence: inhalation, gas exchange and exhalation. When we inhale, the intercostal muscles (between the ribs) contract, increasing the size of the chest cavity and thereby expanding the lungs and drawing air down into the system. Within the lungs, oxygen is extracted from the inhaled air and waste carbon dioxide returned to it. Lastly, exhalation (relaxation of the intercostal muscles) reduces the size of the chest cavity, so forcing the processed air out.

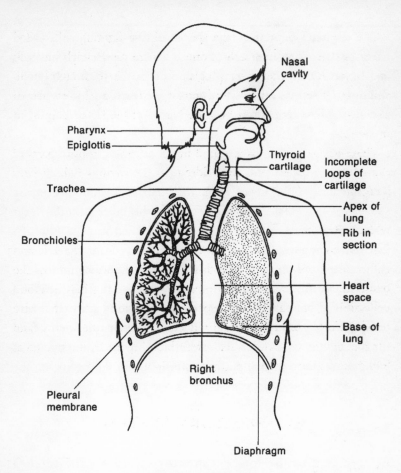

The respiratory system

Each cell in the body needs oxygen to function. The waste products of this process are carbon dioxide and water. Only 20 per cent of inspired air is oxygen, and of that 16 per cent is excreted again during respiration, thus only 4 per cent of available oxygen is absorbed. If the need for oxygen increases, we breathe faster and the heart rate increases, inducing a greater flow of air and thus increased oxygen absorption. An average respiratory rate is 16 breaths each minute.

The respiratory system is best viewed in two parts: the upper and lower systems. The upper part consists of the nasal cavity, pharynx and larynx, while the lower is comprised of the trachea, bronchii and lungs. The lungs themselves encompass the bronchioles, alveoli and pleural membranes.

Upper System

The function of the upper respiratory tract is to humidify, purify and warm the inhaled air, thus enabling the more delicate lower respiratory tract to function satisfactorily. Inhaled air passes through the nasal cavity, which is lined with epithelial cells that filter, warm and moisten the air. The pharynx lies behind and is common to both the respiratory and alimentary tracts. In this area is a collection of lymphatic tissue that is known as the adenoids (these tend to atrophy after childhood). The area between the root of the tongue and the trachea is called the larynx – in men this enlarges at puberty and becomes the Adam's Apple. Within the larynx are the vocal cords; further filtration of the air occurs here.

Lower System

Air passes into the lower respiratory tract via the trachea (windpipe). This is basically a continuation of the larynx, is approximately $4^1/2$ in/$11^1/2$ cm long and made up of 16–20 incomplete loops of cartilage which maintain the airway. The trachea is surrounded by fibrous elastic tissue. At about the level of the fifth thoracic vertebra,. the trachea divides into two bronchii which lead to the lungs and then divide into small bronchioles, which are cartilaginous with elastic walls. The bronchioles divide, reduce in size and terminate in air sacs known as alveoli. This is best envisaged as an inverted tree, with the bronchus as the trunk, bronchioles as the branches and the alveoli as the leaves. The total surface area of the alveoli is approximately 750 sq ft/70 sq m, the average size of a tennis court.

The walls of the trachea, bronchii and bronchioles are lined with minute hairs known as ciliae which produce mucus to maintain a moist environment and also to act as a filter system by trapping dust and foreign particles. By their reflex movement any foreign substance is expelled by coughing or sneezing, in order to prevent impaired function of the delicate alveoli.

Lungs

The basic function of the lungs is to allow a free exchange of gases between the alveoli and the bloodstream. The lungs themselves are conical in shape, the apex at the top. They are separated from each other by the heart and major blood vessels. Each lung is composed of lobes that are extremely well supplied with blood from the pulmonary arteries and veins. These lobes are covered by a double serous membrane known as the pleura. The pleura allow movement without friction from the surrounding rib cage.

The diaphragm and the intercostal muscles contract, thus increasing the thoracic cavity in length. As a result the lungs are stretched, as are the bronchioles and bronchii, and air is drawn down to fill up the increased capacity in the lungs. The diaphragm and the intercostal muscles then relax, causing the rib cage to fall back and forcing the air upwards—thus exhalation occurs.

Between inspiration and exhalation the interchange of gases in the alveoli takes place. Oxygen is passed out into the red blood cells in the capillary network surrounding each alveoli and transported as oxyhaemoglobin in the bloodstream and so to the rest of the body. The carbon dioxide waste is drawn back into the alveoli from the blood, returning to the lungs for reoxygenation.

The blood supply to the lungs is of great importance. Within the lungs, veins carry oxygenated blood and arteries carry deoxygenated blood, contrary to what occurs in other parts of the body. The pulmonary artery conveys blood returning from the body via the heart and to the lungs, for reoxygenation; the pulmonary veins carry blood that is rich with oxygen back to the heart for further pumping to the rest of the body. The arteries enter each lung and branch into arterioles, and further branch to form the capillary network that encases the alveoli. At the capillary level, the exchange of oxygen and carbon dioxide takes place and the capillaries collect to form veins. These veins lead to the pulmonary veins for return to the heart, conveying oxygenated blood for distribution to the body. Expired air is saturated with water vapour, which is at body temperature and, as a consequence, there is a degree of heat loss from the respiratory tract. This heat is released from the body in three ways: through the skin (perspiration), through respiration, and through urination/ defecation.

Respiration is controlled both chemically (the amounts of carbon dioxide and oxygen present in the bloodstream) and by the nervous system (stimulated by a lack of oxygen or an excess of carbon dioxide, it sends a message to the brain that more oxygen is needed); the two reactions are closely linked.

Nervous System

While viewing the systems of the body individually, it is important to remember that each system relies on and is integrated with the others. This monitoring and synchronization is performed through the nervous system.

The nervous system can be considered in two parts: the central nervous system (the brain and spinal cord), at the centre, and the peripheral nervous system, which consists of 31 pairs of nerves and their subdivisions. These nerves leave the spinal cord and branch to all parts of the body.

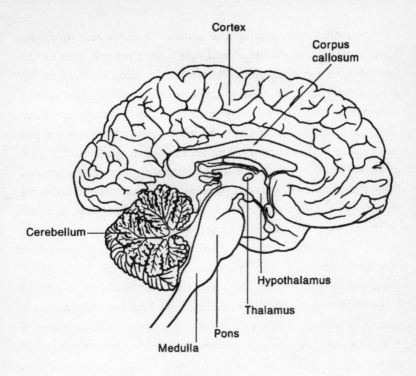

The brain

The Central Nervous System

THE BRAIN

The brain is made up of approximately 12 million nerve cells and weighs around $3^1/_4$ lb/$1^1/_2$ kg. The brain has to be well supplied with oxygen via the blood, to enable these cells to function. Any compromise in the oxygen level can result in serious or fatal consequences, such as a stroke.

The brain is composed of three main areas: the cerebrum, cerebellum, and the brain stem. Each area has specific functions.

The Cerebrum

The cerebrum is made up of two convoluted hemispheres joined by a group of nerve cells, giving the whole a walnut-shaped appearance.

To generalize, each hemisphere of the cerebrum is responsible for control of one half of the body, with communication between hemispheres via the mass of nerve cells joining them. The left hemisphere controls the right side of the body but is also concerned with speech, rationality, logic, analysis and objectivity. The right hemisphere controls the left side of the body and is also concerned with feelings, intuition, subjectivity, imagination and thought. These areas also assess and process all information received from the peripheral nervous system as well as information from the senses, the most complex of all being the interpretation of visual information.

The Cerebellum

The cerebellum, sometimes called the hind brain, is concerned with subconscious control of co-ordination of the skeletal muscle system, enabling accurate, co-ordinated, precise movement. Nerve impulses from the inner ear are processed here to maintain balance.

The Brain Stem

The brain stem links the cerebrum, cerebellum and the spinal cord. It is the main tract for nerve fibres ascending and descending into the spinal cord and has developed as a complicated 'relay point' making connections to and from the cerebrum and, most importantly, controlling vital automatic functions such as heart rate, breathing and consciousness.

THE SPINAL CORD

The spinal cord is the group of nerves of the central nervous system that runs down the body inside the spinal vertebrae. It is about 18 in/46 cm long and the width of a little finger. It is the nervous link between the brain and the organs and outposts of the body, with many nerves branching to relay data to and from the relevant areas.

Both the brain and spinal cord are well protected by the skull and vertebral column. They are surrounded by membranes, the meninges, which contain cerebro-spinal fluid that bathes the delicate structures and acts to absorb shock.

The Peripheral Nervous System

The peripheral nerves consist of elongated nerve cells, called fibres, which have the ability to transmit impulses. These impulses can be sensory (feeling) or motor (command) in nature. These provide two-way communication between the brain and all areas of the body. Nerve fibres have the characteristics of *conductivity* and *irritability*. Conductivity is the ability to transmit impulses. Irritability is the power to respond to stimulation, a process that is partly electrical and partly chemical. Pain, temperature, pressure and touch are all stimuli perceived at the periphery of the body by the sensory nerves. These signals are relayed to the brain, which interprets and responds appropriately. Impulses travel along nerve fibres at an approximate speed of 300 mph.

Nerve cells are extremely delicate, with many intricate connection points between each, and only possess a limited capacity for repair if damaged. Injury, compression, surgery, viral and bacterial infections and lack of oxygen can all cause immense damage to their delicate structures. This damage can impair bodily function.

THE ENDOCRINE SYSTEM

The internal environment of the body is maintained partly by the autonomic nervous system and partly by the endocrine glands. The endocrine glands and the hormones they produce stabilize the body's processes, growth and metabolic rate.

The system consists of a number of glands, widely separated from each other and often referred to as *ductless* glands because the hormones they produce pass directly into the bloodstream. Hormones are basically chemical substances which influence the function of other organs, often in quite different areas of the body. The autonomic nervous system plays a great part in communicating and stimulating these glands to produce and secrete the necessary amounts of hormones to have a stimulatory effect on other organs.

The following list shows the glands, some singly, some in pairs, which make up the endocrine system. Of these glands, the pineal alone remains a mystery: no one knows its exact function.

- 1 Pituitary
- 1 Thyroid
- 4 Parathyroid
- 2 Adrenal
- Islets of Langerhans (in pancreas)
- 1 Thymus
- 2 Testes (male)
- 2 Ovaries (female)
- 1 Pineal

The Pituitary Gland

The main operator of the endocrine system is the *pituitary*, which is the size of a pea and is situated at the base of the brain, being responsible for nine different hormones. Some of these hormones stimulate other endocrine glands into action, yet the pituitary constantly acts as a feedback monitor for the whole system, responding to the level of concentration in the bloodstream of hormones produced by other glands and adjusting its output of stimulating hormone accordingly. The pituitary, however, falls under the direct influence of the hypothalamus of the brain situated just above the pituitary. The hypothalamus produces stimulating and inhibitory hormones in response to impulses received in the brain; these pass the short distance to the pituitary to enable it to respond by increasing or decreasing its secretory activity. The *growth hormone*, produced by the pituitary, effects mainly the development of the skeleton. Thyroid, adrenal, gonadotrophic (concerned with ovaries and testes) and lactogenic (concerned with production of breastmilk) stimulating hormones are also produced by the pituitary. In co-operation with the hypothalamus, the pituitary forms a functional unit responsible for the production of vasopressin (anti-diuretic hormone) which regulates the amounts of water excreted by the kidneys, and also oxytocin, responsible for milk stimulation and contraction of the uterus following childbirth.

The Thyroid Gland

The thyroid gland is situated in the neck, at the base of the cervical vertebrae. It has two connecting lobes, is extremely vascular and of all of the glands has the highest failure rate. Hormones produced here require the presence of iodine, taken from the bloodstream; any excess of iodine is stored for future use. Satisfactory mental and physical development, maintenance of healthy skin and hair, nerve stability and control of the utilization of oxygen are due to the action of this gland. Over-activity of this gland causes *thyrotoxicosis* (speeded up metabolic rate); under-activity causes *myxodema* (sluggish metabolic rate).

The Parathyroid Glands

The parathyroids are in two pairs. They are only a $1/2$ in/$2/3$cm long and lie at the posterior part of the thyroid. They are responsible for maintaining the correct calcium levels in the blood.

The Adrenals

The adrenal glands sit on top of the kidneys. They are constructed of a cortex (outer) and medulla (inner), each of which has entirely different functions. Three main groups of hormones are produced from cholesterol in the body by the cortex. *Cortisone* and *hydrocortisone* regulate the carbohydrate metabolism. *Aldosterone* influences the reabsorption and excretion of salts in the kidneys and maintains water balance. Sex hormones (androgens and oestrogens) are also produced by the adrenals. These hormones influence the development and maintenance of secondary sexual characteristics.

The medulla (inner area) of the adrenals produces adrenaline and nor-adrenaline ('fight or flight' hormones) in response to stimulation from the nervous system.

Islets of Langerhans

In the pancreas lie groups of cells known as the Islets of Langerhans which have an important role in the production of glucagon and insulin, influenced by the glucose level of the bloodstream. Glucagon mobilizes glycogen stores in the liver to be absorbed into the bloodstream, thus increasing the blood sugar level in response to low blood sugar (due to insufficient carbohydrate intake or excessive exercise). Insulin has the opposite effect, reducing blood sugar level by encouraging cells to absorb glucose from the blood supply. If the cells producing insulin cease to function or are diseased, diabetes ensues.

The Thymus

The thymus gland lies within the thoracic cavity. It is active during childhood but diminishes during adolescence and fibroses (shrivels and becomes harder) in adulthood. Its functions are not entirely clear, but is thought to be concerned with the production of lymphocytes and may be associated with the development of secondary sexual characteristics, hence its atrophy after puberty.

The Testes and Ovaries

The major androgen (masculinizing hormone–testosterone) producer in the male is the testes. In the female the ovaries produce oestrogen and progesterone, which control fertility and the menstrual cycle.

REPRODUCTIVE SYSTEM

Female

The function of the female reproductive system is to form an ovum (egg), which, if fertilized by a sperm from the male, needs a safe place to be nurtured and nourished until it is capable of independent existence. The system is comprised of two ovaries, a pair of Fallopian tubes, the uterus and the vagina.

During the years from puberty to the menopause a woman ovulates at monthly intervals, approximately 400 times. If the egg is not fertilized then the lining of the womb is shed and menstruation occurs. The endocrine glands are responsible for this cycle–the hypothalamus, the pituitary and the ovaries.

The Ovaries

The ovaries are almond-shaped, about $1^{1}/_{2}$ in/4 cm long. They lie in the pelvic basin. At birth, they contain millions of immature eggs housed inside follicles, but only a percentage of these reach maturity. At puberty the ovaries are stimulated by hormones from the pituitary gland: the follicle stimulating hormone (FSH) and the leutenising hormone (LH). Secondary sexual characteristics are also developing in the rest of the body at this time, for example breast enlargement.

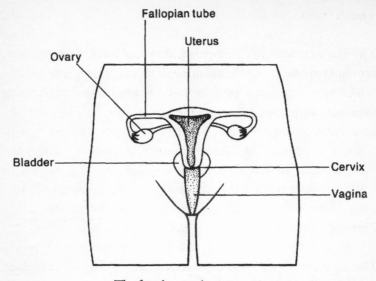

The female reproductive system

After puberty, each month a follicle in the ovary is stimulated by the FSH from the pituitary, causing it to grow and produce oestrogen, while the ovum develops within it. Only one ovum fully matures during the cycle even though several others may start to mature. The follicle ruptures, releasing the ovum (ovulation) into the peritoneal cavity close to the free end of the Fallopian tube. The follicle meanwhile comes under the influence of LH and turns into a 'yellow body' which then starts secreting progesterone. The level of progesterone is highest after ovulation in order to stimulate the endometrium (lining of the uterus) to prepare for the implantation of the egg. The ovum passes down the Fallopian tube and into the uterus. If the egg is not fertilized, the LH from the pituitary is inhibited; this then has a knock-on effect in decreasing the production of progesterone from the yellow body and causes it to degenerate. Due to falling levels of progesterone menstruation occurs, i.e. the lining of the uterus is shed as it is not required.

The Uterus

The uterus is a thick, muscular, hollow pear-shaped organ lying between the bladder and the rectum. The narrow neck at the base is the *cervix*, which juts into the top of the vagina. Opening into each side of the rounded top of the uterus are the Fallopian tubes. Each Fallopian tube is about 4 in/10 cm long, with a free funnel-shaped end opening into the peritoneum, close to the ovaries but without direct contact. The function of the Fallopian tubes is to transport ova from the ovaries to the uterus by means of tiny waving hair-like structures that waft the ova towards the uterus. Fertilization usually takes place in the Fallopian tubes.

The uterus consists of three layers: the outer layer (the *peritoneum*) which covers the body of the uterus, the *myometrium* (the thick muscular wall), and an inner lining called the *endometrium*. The main function of the uterus is to nourish and protect the fertilized ovum and later, by muscular activity, to allow the fully developed foetus to be born.

The Vagina

The vagina is approximately 4 in/10 cm long and lies in front of the rectum but behind the urethra. It is fibro muscular and lined with a mucous membrane. There are a number of friendly micro-organisms present which are responsible for maintaining the correct pH balance (slightly acidic) that prevents infection both locally and from spreading upwards towards the uterus. The vagina opens at the vulva, the collective term for the inner and outer labia and clitoris.

The Breasts

The breasts (mammary glands) are accessory glands of the female system, developing at puberty and consisting of glandular, fibrous and fatty tissue. The fatty tissue which lies between the glandular lobes determines the size and shape of the breasts. The glandular lobes are able to produce milk in the event of childbirth, being stimulated by hormone production from the pituitary. Ducts leading from the milk-producing glands converge at the nipple.

Male

The male reproductive system consists basically of two testes, associated glands and a series of ducts, all of which open at the tip of the penis. Although the male urethra is significantly longer than the female and thus less prone to urinary infections, because the prostate, testes and other ducts open directly into it, this does mean that urinary infections can easily spread to the reproductive organs.

The Testes

The testes are almond-shaped and usually descend during infancy into the *scrotum* (the muscular pouch of skin behind the penis). The reason they lie outside the body is that for the satisfactory production of sperm the temperature has to be cooler than body temperature. The testes manufacture sperm and produce the male sex hormone, testosterone, under the influence of the leutenising hormone from the pituitary. Testosterone is absorbed directly into the blood supply and is required for the development of the male reproductive system, the 'breaking' of the voice at puberty and the growth of body and facial hair, and also for the production of sperm.

It takes about 60–70 days for a sperm to mature; approximately 10–30 thousand million are produced per month. The function of the sperm, if introduced into the female reproductive tract, is to fertilize the ovum and thus produce a zygote which grows and divides to form an embryo and ultimately a new human being.

Inside each testis is a mass of coiled tubes called the *epididymis* where the sperm mature and from whence they pass to the *vas deferens* and seminal vesicles for storage.

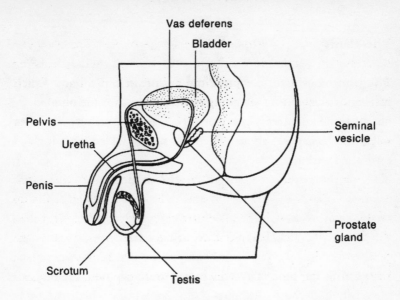

The male reproductive system

The Seminal Vesicles

The seminal vesicles are two pouches found behind the bladder which secrete a sticky, sugary fluid from which the sperm are nourished and gain their mobility. The ejaculatory ducts lead from each vesicle into the prostate to join the urethra. During ejaculation the seminal vesicles and the prostate gland contract strongly and expel the semen into the urethra and out of the end of the penis. If mature sperm are not ejaculated, they disintegrate and are re-absorbed into the body.

The Prostate

The prostate gland lies below the bladder and around the top of the urethra. It is approximately the size and shape of a chestnut. Secretions of acids, trace elements and enzymes are added to the semen by the prostate to help activate the sperm.

Frequently in old age, the prostate enlarges and hardens and can give rise to problems with urinating.

The Penis

The penis consists of a root in the perineum and a body which surrounds the urethra. It contains erectile tissue, surrounded by fibrous tissue and deeply pigmented skin. At its extremity is an area called the *glans penis*, above which the skin is folded onto itself to form the foreskin.

DIGESTIVE SYSTEM

Digestion is the process by which food materials are changed both physically and chemically into a substance from which the body can absorb nutrients. It is best viewed as a four-part system: ingestion, digestion, absorption and elimination.

Ingestion

Food, when taken into the mouth, is masticated by the teeth and moved around by the tongue. Saliva is released and mixes with the food. The enzymes contained in saliva begin the digestive process. The prepared food then enters the oesophagus and travels to the stomach, propelled by rhythmic contractions of the muscular walls (the *peristaltic wave*). The oesophagus is the narrowest part of the digestive system.

Digestion

When the prepared food enters the stomach it is churned, causing further mechanical breakdown, while being mixed with gastric juice. The gastric juice is secreted from the stomach walls and contains hydrochloric acid and further enzymes, as well as mucus. Both the hydrochloric acid and the enzymes start the breakdown of

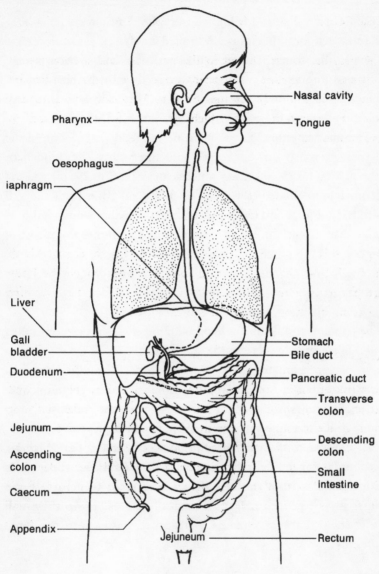

The digestive system

proteins into more soluble compounds. The mucus lines the stomach and prevents damage from the acid.

The food, once churned and mixed with the gastric juice,

becomes paste-like and is known as *chyme*. This chyme remains in the stomach for a short time. A limited amount of absorption takes place in the stomach: water, glucose, alcohol and some drugs are absorbed through the walls and pass directly into the bloodstream. The chyme is slowly released from the stomach into the small intestine through the pyloric sphincter.

The small intestine, despite its name, is the longest section of the digestive tract. It can be divided into three parts: the duodenum (the first 10 in/25 cm), the jejunum, (the next 8 ft/2½ m) and the ileum (approximately the final 12 ft/3½ m). Bile from the gall bladder and juices from the pancreas enter the duodenum and help neutralize the acid from the stomach and continue the digestive process.

Absorption

The jejunum and ileum are lined with finger-like projections called *villi*. These greatly increase the surface of the small intestine to an area of approximately 200 sq ft/19 sq m. The villi contain a network of blood and lymph vessels, and have extremely thin walls to enable the absorption of nutrients from the processed food through the intestine and into the blood and lymph.

At the base of the villi are collections of lymph nodes which are responsible for the destruction of micro-organisms. Intestinal juices from glands within the cell walls are secreted to complete the digestion of proteins, fats and carbohydrates. From the small intestine, whatever remains unabsorbed passes into the large intestine.

THE LIVER

The nutrients absorbed into the bloodstream through the villi are transported via the hepatic portal vein to the liver for metabolism. The liver is the most versatile organ of the body. It acts as a chemical factory where raw materials are broken down, stored and then dispatched when required. Fats, surplus carbohydrates and amino acids are converted into glycogen for storage; this glycogen can be readily reconverted into glucose when required. Unwanted nitrogenous material from the metabolism of proteins is converted into urea. The formation of plasma proteins, the production of antibodies and antitoxins and blood-clotting agents also take place here. Vitamins A, B and D are stored until required, as is iron (derived from the diet and from the breakdown of old red blood cells in the spleen).

Elimination

The remaining unabsorbed food, used digestive juices and bacteria pass to the large intestine, which is approximately 5 ft/1½ m long and has a larger diameter than the small intestine. At this stage the material is fairly liquid. During its passage through the large intestine, water, minerals and some drugs are absorbed very slowly into the bloodstream, rendering the contents semi-solid faeces. The peristaltic contractions by which food passes through the digestive system are slower here. The time taken for material to pass through depends on the amount of roughage in the diet. The faeces are collected in the lower part of the large intestine and the rectum to be periodically expelled via the anus.

Urinary System

The urinary system is basically a process of filtration and excretion. The other excretory systems of the body are the skin, lungs and liver. The body's surplus water and chemical waste is processed from the blood by the kidneys and excreted from the body as urine. The liver combines toxic ammonia, produced by the metabolism of proteins within the body, with carbon dioxide to

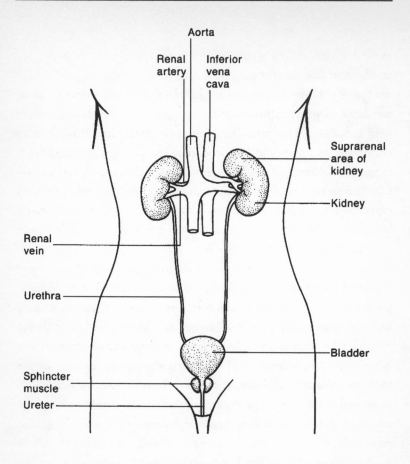

The urinary system

produce the less poisonous urea, which is removed from the blood by the kidneys. The minimum urinary output required to remove waste products from the body is 1 pint/500 ml per day, but generally a healthy adult will pass between 2-3 pints/1-1¹/₂ litres a day.

The urinary system comprises two kidneys, two ureters, the bladder and the urethra. The kidneys lie in the posterior part of the abdomen, one on each side of the spine. The right kidney is usually lower than the left, due to the considerable amount of space taken up by the liver. Each is approximately 4¹/₂ in/11¹/₂ cm long by 2–3 in/5–7$\frac{1}{2}$ cm wide. They are delicate but well protected and held in place by fatty tissue.

The kidneys are connected to the bladder by the ureters, which are about 11 in/28 cm in length.

The bladder is a reservoir for collecting the urine before excretion. Its size is variable depending on the amount of urine it happens to contain. Normally the bladder allows 10$\frac{1}{2}$ fl oz/300 ml of urine to be collected before emptying; nerves within its walls signal when it is full. The urine is then discharged from the body via the urethra, which is 6–7 in/15–18 cm long in men but only 1–1$\frac{1}{2}$ in/2$\frac{1}{2}$–4 cm long in women.

The function of the kidneys is to maintain the internal water and chemical balance of the body. The blood carries many substances, some of which are necessary, some desirable in only precisely limited quantities, and others that are harmful. The kidneys monitor the volume, acidity, toxicity and mineral content of the blood every 30 minutes and ensure that the correct balance of the blood is maintained. Blood pressure is controlled via hormones produced by the kidneys. The manufacture of red blood cells in the bone marrow is stimulated from here, and vitamin D is also activated.

The kidney is enveloped by a fatty capsule and consists of an outer area called the cortex and an inner part called the medulla. The renal artery enters the kidney and then branches into more than a million minute capillaries. The capillaries twist and twine into a knot called the *glomerulus*; each glomerulus is encased by a capsule called Bowman's capsule. This capsule in turn leads to a coiling tubule that joins up with others of the same and eventually leads to the ureter. Together the glomerulus and the Bowman's capsule form a microscopic filter-bed called the Malpighian body.

The capillary entry into the glomerulus is smaller than the exit, consequently the blood is forced through at high pressure. The pressure forces fluid out through the walls of the glomerulus into the Bowman's capsule. The fluid after this filtration is largely water, urea, mineral salts, glucose and some toxins. However, because of the size of the filter pores, red and white blood cells, plasma and proteins remain in the capillary. The filtered fluid then runs from the Bowman's capsule into the twisted tubule, which is surrounded by a network of capillaries that branch from the single capillary taking the filtered blood away from the glomerulus. It is here, in the second part of the process, that selective reabsorption takes place.

Selective reabsorption is the method by which the useful contents of the fluid from the Bowman's capsule are soaked up and passed back into the bloodstream via the renal vein. These include some 99 per cent of the water, all the glucose and the precise quantity of mineral salts to fulfil the body's current requirements. After selective reabsorption the remaining liquid, now called urine, is collected in the centre of the kidney and passes down the ureters into the bladder.

Urine itself is sterile. It is composed of approximately 96 per cent water; urea and salts form the other 4 per cent. During the summer or when hot, more surplus water is excreted through the skin as cooling perspiration. In a temperate climate this is normally 500–750 ml/1–1½ pints a day but can be very much higher – as much as 1½ litres/3 pints an hour – when exercising on a very hot day. This is why a smaller, more concentrated amount of urine is produced at these times.

THE SKIN

The skin is the body's largest organ. Stretched out, it would cover between 15 and 20 sq ft/1½–2 sq m. It is semi-permeable and one of the most active organs of the body. Among the skin's functions are the control of body temperature, sensing the outside world by means of the numerous nerve endings, insulation and protection of the body from organic invasion and injury, vitamin-D manufacture and the secretion of some substances and absorption of others.

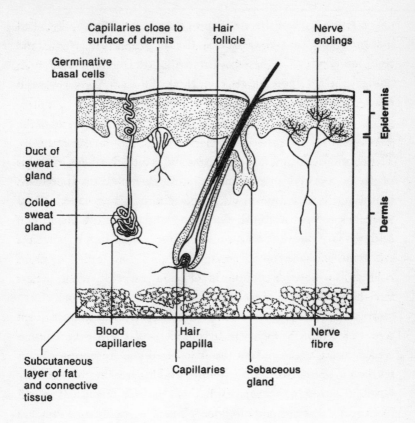

A section of skin

The skin is composed of two layers: the outer layer (the epidermis) and the lower layer (the dermis).

The Epidermis

The epidermis itself is made up of layers. The outer layer of the epidermis is composed of dead cells. New cells are produced at the lower level and continually push the older cells upwards. By the time these cells reach the surface level they are dead. Normally, these dead cells slough off, although in some places they continue to form a fibrous layer, as on the heels of the feet and parts of the hand. The epidermis has no blood supply but the lower layer contains lymph supplied from the dermis to provide nourishment.

The lower level of the epidermis contains specialized cells called melanoblasts, which produce the pigment melanin. This colouration protects the body from the ultra-violet radiation in sunlight and is responsible for the colour of the skin. Hair roots and sweat gland ducts pass through the epidermis.

The Dermis

The dermis lies below the epidermis and is a thicker layer made up largely of connective tissue, making it tough and elastic. It contains blood and lymphatic vessels, nerve endings, hair follicles and sebaceous and sweat glands. The blood vessels are in the form of a fine capillary network and the lymphatic vessels supply nutrients and drain the epidermis above.

There is a wide distribution of different types of sensory nerve endings in the dermis, each designed to deal with the one of five distinct senses: touch, contact, heat, cold, pressure and pain. Each type of receptor is stimulated by one particular sensation. Pain, as well as being registered by the specialized pain receptors, is also registered by the many 'free' nerve endings which are unevenly distributed close to the epidermal layer and respond to all stimuli that affect the other specialized receptors. The sensation of pain acts as a vital warning system, preventing further damage. For example, the reflex action of dropping something hot before it burns. Pain also occurs when any of the receptors is over-stimulated.

Hair roots are anchored in this layer. Each hair is composed of two parts: the root and the shaft. The shaft grows up through the epidermis to the surface. A cluster of cells at the base form a bulb, which is housed in a follicle. The bulb produces new hair cells that push up the older cells along the follicle, which die, change into keratin and become part of the shaft, emerging from the epidermis as hair. Sebaceous glands housed in the hair follicle secrete sebum, which lubricates and is carried to the surface by the hair. Sebum acts to keep skin supple and waterproof and, being bactericidal, prevents invasion by micro-organisms present on the surface. Hair colour is governed by its melanin content (white hair, therefore, contains no melanin).

Body Temperature

The skin plays an important role in maintaining the correct body temperature. This is achieved through activity of the sweat glands and blood vessels. When body temperature rises the sweat glands release more sweat to evaporate from the skin, so cooling it. The blood vessels dilate to carry more blood near the surface to be cooled.

Vitamin D

A fatty substance present in sebum is affected by the action of ultra-violet rays in sunlight; this substance and the ultra-violet rays combine to produce vitamin D. The vitamin D thus formed is absorbed into the bloodstream and utilized within the body, ensuring the satisfactory uptake and metabolism of calcium.

MUSCULO-SKELETAL SYSTEM

Our posture, ability to move freely and perform many complicated manoeuvres is due to our possession of a wonderfully engineered system of bones, muscles, ligaments, joints and connective tissue, which also serves to keep our vital organs separate. This system is required to be both simultaneously rigid and flexible.

The skeleton has three basic functions: to support and give shape to our soft body tissues; to allow the attachment of muscles which can pull the bones into different positions, causing them to act as

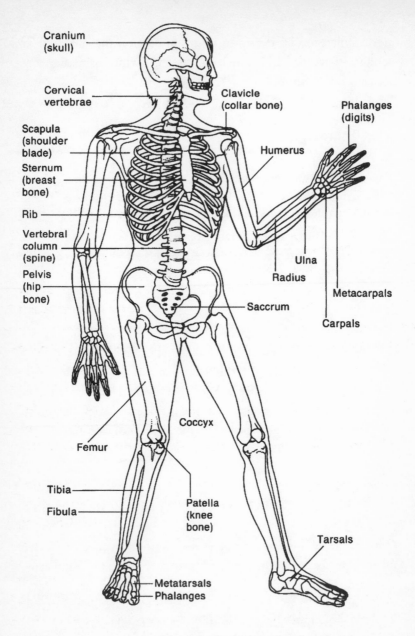

The skeletal system

levers (this translates into movement); and to offer protection to vital organs, many of which are extremely delicate.

The Bones

Bone is made of living tissue, which is constantly being renewed or removed. Skeletons are renewed many times during a lifetime, in response to stress and load. There are two distinct types of bone which constitute the framework of the skeleton and which have developed in response to their function. *Compact bone* is hard and dense, forming the surface layer of all bones and the tubular shafts of long bones. *Cancellous bone* is honeycombed in structure, lighter yet extremely strong, containing the bone marrow which produces red blood corpuscles.

The **skull** (cranium) consists of eight different bones fused together by sutures, the development of which is incomplete until the age of 18 months, hence the need for extreme care with babies. The cranium forms an extremely effective shield for the delicate brain within. The face comprises some 14 bones, the jaw bone (mandible) being the strongest and only movable bone of the skull.

The **vertebral column** consists of 24 separate and movable bones, plus the sacrum (five fused bones) and the coccyx (four fused bones). These vertebrae are divided into groups depending upon their position: 7 cervical, 12 thoracic and 5 lumbar. Each vertebra has a central hole to allow the passage of the spinal cord; it has developed to protect this vital, delicate structure. Due to the number of individual bones there is a certain amount of movement possible through the spine. It acts as a support for the skull and forms the axis of the trunk, having attached to it the ribs and sternum, shoulder girdle, pelvic girdle and lower limbs.

The **sacrum** has five fused vertebrae which link with the

innominate bones to form the pelvic girdle, which has two sockets into which the heads of the femurs (thigh bones) sit. The female pelvis is wider and shallower than the male, being adapted for childbirth.

The **thoracic cage**, as its name implies, is a protective cage for the organs and systems of the chest (lungs, heart) and consists of the sternum (breastbone), 12 pairs of ribs and 12 thoracic vertebrae. The **shoulder girdle** is made up of the clavicle (collar bone) and scapulae (shoulder blades), to which is linked the humerus (upper arm).

THE JOINTS

Where bones meet in the body there are joints, which are classified by the amount of movement possible between the articulating surfaces: there are fixed, cartilaginous and synovial joints. The ends of all bones are protected by very smooth cartilage to prevent friction.

Fixed joints allow no movement, the articular surfaces being joined by tough fibrous tissue and frequently the edges of the bones being dovetailed into each other, as in the case of the sutures of the skull.

Cartilaginous joints allow only slight movement. A wad of cartilage lying between the ends of each bone acts as a shock absorber. The intervertebral discs are cartilaginous joints.

Synovial joints are variously movable, movement being dictated by the shape of the articulating surfaces. These joints are enclosed by a capsule of tough fibrous tissue whose inner cells produce synovial fluid, to act as shock absorber and lubricant. These joints tend to be at weight-bearing points, such as at the shoulder, elbow, hip, knee, pelvis and sacrum.

Different types of synovial joint allow differing amounts of movement. The ball and socket joints (such as those of the shoulder or hip) offer the greatest movement (for rotation of arms and legs). Hinge joints allow movement in one plane only – as is possible at the elbow, knee, ankle or fingers. Sliding joints allow the articular

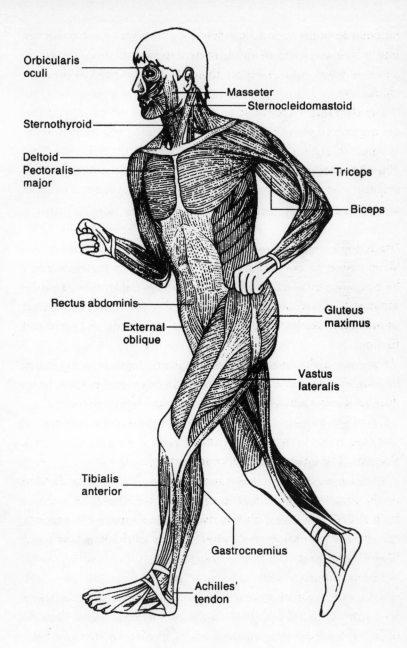

Orbicularis oculi

Masseter
Sternocleidomastoid

Sternothyroid

Deltoid
Pectoralis major

Triceps

Biceps

Rectus abdominis

Gluteus maximus

External oblique

Vastus lateralis

Tibialis anterior

Gastrocnemius

Achilles' tendon

Muscles of the body

surfaces to glide over each other – e.g. the vertebrae, wrists and ankles. Pivot joints allow movement around one axis only, for example rotational – the atlas and axis bones at the top of the neck. Lastly, saddle joints allow movement around two axes – e.g. the fingers and toes.

The Muscles

Movement of any joint is produced by the contraction and relaxation of muscles attached to the bones on each side of the joint. These muscles are made up of a fleshy part and a tendonous part. Generally, the tendonous part is attached to the bone and is fairly inelastic, thus keeping the joint within stable limits. In order to produce movement at a joint, a muscle or its tendon must stretch across the joint. As a muscle contracts, it shortens and pulls, thus acting as a lever. The muscles of the skeleton are arranged in pairs or groups, some being antagonistic towards others. Our muscle tone is important as it enables us to maintain correct posture. In the case of moving an individual joint, one muscle has to contract and its antagonist muscle must relax. In performing finer, more complicated tasks, e.g. writing, there is a complicated co-ordination of many muscles.

Many muscles have complicated names associated with their shape – such as the deltoid muscle, so-called because it is shaped like the Greek letter D – or with the number of points of attachment (e.g. the biceps), or the names of the bones to which they are attached.

Ligaments attach bone to bone, to maintain stability, but possess no contractile power. One can easily understand that this system as a whole, with its series of complicated interactions between muscles, tendons, ligaments and bones, enables us to move freely and maintain posture. One can also see how everyday stresses, strains and injury which can accumulate over the years could not

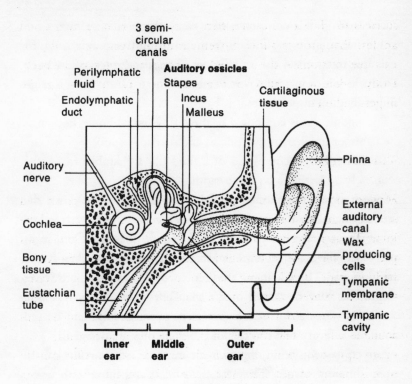

3 semi-
circular
canals

Auditory ossicles
Stapes
Incus
Malleus

Perilymphatic
fluid

Endolymphatic
duct

Cartilaginous
tissue

Auditory
nerve

Pinna

Cochlea

External
auditory
canal

Wax
producing
cells

Bony
tissue

Eustachian
tube

Tympanic
membrane

Tympanic
cavity

Inner
ear

Middle
ear

Outer
ear

The ear

only severely compromise our freedom to move and perform basic
tasks but might also have more far-reaching effects on our general
levels of health.

THE SPECIAL SENSES

Hearing

The ear consists of three distinct parts: the outer, middle and inner
ears.

The outer ear is composed of a cartilaginous flap (pinna) from which the auditory canal leads to the eardrum (tympanum), which seals the outer from the middle ear. The auditory canal is lined with cells which produce wax to protect the eardrum from foreign bodies that might penetrate it.

The middle ear is composed of three tiny linked bones known as the hammer (malleus), anvil (incus) and stirrup (stapes).

The inner ear is comprised of a fluid-filled chamber called the cochlea lying within a bony labyrinth.

Sound waves are collected by the pinna and funnelled down the auditory canal to the eardrum. The eardrum, a tightly stretched membrane, vibrates in sympathy to the sound it receives and in its turn causes the hammer, anvil and stirrup to amplify the vibrations to the inner ear. The vibrations are then converted into pressure waves within the fluid contained in the snail-like spirals of the cochlea. Here, the waves are sensed by receptive nerve endings and relayed along the auditory nerve to the brain, where they are decoded.

Also contained within the inner ear are three semi-circular canals, set in different planes. They are fluid-filled and lined with nerve endings. Movement of the head causes the fluid to move against the nerve endings and so, by comparing the differing impulses from the various canals and computing this information with data from the eyes and the rest of the body, the brain is informed of our position in space and gives the sense of balance. An infection of this part of the ear gives rise to dizziness and nausea, which is made worse by continued movement. Because of its proximity to the brain, any ear infection should be taken seriously.

Linking the middle ear to the throat (nasopharynx) is the eustachian tube. This allows the equalization of pressure on both sides of the eardrum by admitting or releasing air. If the pressure is not equal – for instance if the eustachian tube is blocked by catarrh or by a sudden change in altitude – the ear drum is sucked in and ceases to vibrate satisfactorily. When the pressure is equalized the ear drum 'pops'.

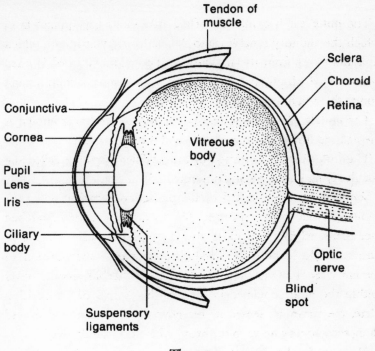

The eye

Sight

The eye is basically a jelly-filled sphere, the walls of which consist of three layers.

The outer layer forms the white of the eye and maintains the eye's shape and form; it is called the sclera. The front area of the sclera is transparent and forms the cornea.

The central layer is the choroid. This layer is extremely vascular and pigmented to prevent the loss of light; it can be seen through the cornea as the iris. The aperture in the iris is called the pupil.

The inner layer, where the light-sensitive cells are found, is the retina. These light-sensitive cells are called rods and cones.

The eye's lens lies behind the iris, with the space between filled with a watery substance called aqueous humour. The rest of the eye is filled with the more jelly-like vitreous humour. The cornea is covered by a protective film called the conjunctiva, which is cleansed and lubricated by bactericidal fluid produced by the tear glands. The ciliary muscle adjusts the shape of the lens and so bends the light to focus the image on the retina. The amount of light entering the eye is controlled by the pupil, which is dilated or constricted by the muscles of the iris.

Light, reflected from an object, passes through the cornea which bends the rays through the pupil to the lens. This brings the light

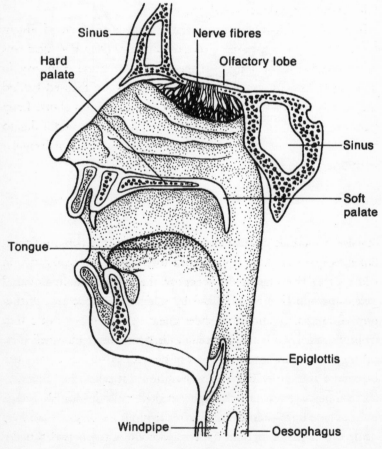

The organs of smell and taste

to focus on the retina. The retina consists of millions of light-sensitive rods and cones. The rods are the most sensitive but register only black and white, while the cones register colour but need more light to do so. Consequently, in dim light we experience only monochrome vision. The cones are of three types, each registering red, green or blue light. These impulses are then transmitted to the brain via the optic nerve. The brain then has to decipher these impulses and form them into the image we see. It receives two images, which are very small, upside down, in two dimensions and only in three colours; it then forms them into the full-colour, three-dimensional image we see.

In short-sightedness (myopia) distant objects are focused just in front of the retina, resulting in poor definition. Defective ligaments or an eye that is too long in shape can be the cause. Similarly, in long-sightedness (hypermetropia) near objects are focused behind the retina, due to lazy muscles or the eye being too short. Long sight can become more marked with age (presbyopia) and is due to loss of elasticity of the lens. Astigmatism is the result of irregular curvature of the cornea.

Smell

Smell is a more acute sense than taste, although the two are linked. Smell receptors are located in the olfactory area of the nasal cavity, in the roof of the nose. The receptors have fine mucus-covered extensions which are stimulated by molecules in the air. During normal breathing some molecules reach the receptors, but a sniff transmits more molecules and causes identification of the smell. The odour molecules are dissolved in the mucus which covers the extensions and the information relayed to the receptors and passed to the brain. We quickly lose our awareness of individual smells, which can have dangerous consequences (as in the case of gas – we may notice it at first but then become oblivious to it, and thus be poisoned). A trained nose can distinguish thousands of different smells.

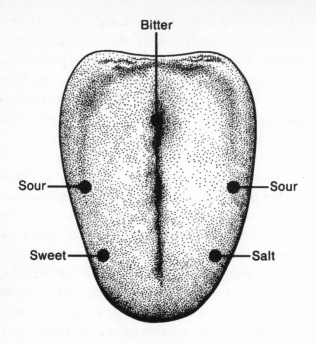

The taste buds

Taste

Taste is a chemical process and requires a substance to be dissolved in either saliva or water before it can be registered. The surface of the tongue is covered in tiny projections, known as papillae, in which the taste buds are embedded. There are approximately 2000 taste buds which are sensitive to only four basic tastes: sweet, sour, salt and bitter. The taste buds are unevenly distributed over the tongue – the sweet and salt receptors at the front, sour receptors at the sides, and bitterness receptors at the back. The bitterness receptors are the most sensitive, the sweet ones the least. Impulses from these receptors are transmitted to the taste area of the brain and interpreted.

Taste and flavour are not the same. Flavour involves the sense of smell as well as taste. As we eat, constituents of the food waft up through the nose to the olfactory area and are registered, so a food's flavour is a combination of its taste and smell. When the nose is blocked, as with a heavy cold, the smell receptors cannot receive information about the food being consumed, therefore only the taste buds receive stimulation and it becomes difficult to distinguish between foods of a similar texture; hence we seem to lose our sense of taste as well.

It is hoped that this brief overview of the systems of the body has demonstrated how they are all inextricably connected, and that this has made you more aware of and sensitive to the complex functioning of your body, the nature of ill health and the various steps that may be required to correct it.

The remainder of the book, detailing the natural therapies and individual practitioners' interpretations of them, will try to address not just the specific complaint you have but set it in a wider context and examine all its interrelated aspects as it affects you as a *whole being*.

PART THREE

THE THERAPIES

❧ ACUPRESSURE ❧

JOSKA RAMELOW

The supreme TAO is imperceptible
its changes and transformations
are endless.

HUANG DI NEI JING, 'SU WEN'

ORIGINS

The law of *change* has been pronounced the only certainty in an otherwise constantly changing world by Chinese mystics and medics alike. Great changes have certainly taken place in the medical world in a space of only the last 100 years, with the introduction of ever-more powerful microscopes coupled with an unquenchable thirst for more discoveries beyond the boundaries of our ordinary senses. Successful transplantations fuelled the drive to unravel the mysteries of the genetic structures of Creation. Until a short while ago we thought the light at the end of the tunnel was getting brighter and that, soon, devastating diseases like cancer, chronic degenerative problems such as rheumatoid arthritis and other painful physical suffering could be eradicated for good.

The specialization, however, that led us to believe this was imminent divorced us from seeing the complexities in our everyday lives unheard of at the turn of the century. Our lives are surrounded by potentially harmful materials inside and outside our homes and at our workplaces. The invention of plastic has produced thousands of applications in our environment without which these words could not have been typed, for instance. Our bodies have become charged up with static electricity and our food bombarded with microwave technology, if we have opted for the 'blessings' of a modern lifestyle. Thousands of synthetic colourants and flavour enhancers spice our food, which ultimately adds more to the problems.

We have chosen to look at our lives in a manner that tends to break down and analyse everything into fragments of fragments. As useful as this may be in the pursuit of understanding the microscopic and subatomic building-plan, we have forgotten the whole, with its own methodology of asking holistic questions concerning our health and well-being.

Absence of ease generates *Dis-ease*, which can go unnoticed before our contemporary understanding of disease diagnoses pathological changes of the tissue requiring medical attention. The big 'buzzword' of our day is 'Stress', highlighting this absence of ease or equilibrium necessary to maintain a productive and healthy lifestyle.

PHILOSOPHY

The theory of Chinese medicine is the same for Acupressure, Acupuncture, Herbalism and other disciplines because it centres around the study of a person as a whole, bearing in mind the prime question of how to maintain a lifestyle full of vitality and in harmony with the environmental forces. All the *stems* and *branches* of Chinese medicine are based on the ancient classics, one of which is the *Huang Di Nei Jing*, a collection of discussions on health and related subjects between the Yellow Emperor and his court physician Chi Po, dating back 25 centuries.

The following conversation is recorded in its 'Su Wen' section, on the subject of how to preserve and maintain vigour and health.

The Yellow Emperor wonders why men of high antiquity were able to live 100 years without impairment to their ability to move and act. In contrast, he states his puzzlement that contemporary man should only live to half that age, and speculates whether the times have changed or man simply lost his longevity. To this Chi Po replies,

The men of antiquity understood the TAO (life). They therefore strove to adapt their existence to the rules of YIN and YANG and to live in harmony with numerical calculations. Moderation determined the consumption of food and drink. They arose and slept in accordance with a consistent order. No one depleted his strength through unseemly behaviour. Thus men of antiquity preserved both body and mind with their full powers and reached the full extent of life accorded by Nature. The men of today are totally different. They prepare their soup with wine, and unseemly behaviour has become the rule. They intoxicate themselves...and in gratifying their carnal appetites, they deplete the essence of their existence. They strive mightily to give pleasure to the heart, yet they conduct their lives contrary to the goals of true happiness.

Just looking at oneself or around one's own circle of friends today these words seem to carry a lot of weight, and one wonders to what extent real evolution of humanity's condition has brought about changes that would set us far apart from those men of antiquity. One has to remember that these were not words uttered as moral injunction; on the contrary, they were observations based on the study of man and how to preserve as much energy and nourishment internally in order to gain a long life and happy fulfilment.

The strategies towards this end were composed of graded responses to the needs of the particular person looking for help. For that reason non-invasive techniques like massage, meditation, exercise and diet, for instance, were preferred to the more crisis-oriented techniques like Acupuncture and Herbalism. Even Acupuncture and Herbalism are still firmly rooted in the field that has come to be known by the term 'preventative medicine'.

Because our understanding of disease is not as refined as the Oriental viewpoint, our medical perception is exclusively geared towards real crisis that can be called cancer, diabetes, rheumatoid arthritis, etc., usually all conditions where the balance in the body has been upset for a long time and pathological changes have set in.

Massage, particularly, is up to this day the most joyful way of receiving a real treat because it contains elements of detoxification, relaxation and rejuvenation which, taken together on a regular basis, are able truly to work in a preventative way, boosting immunity, relieving stress and strengthening internal energy levels.

THEORY IN PRACTICE

The Acupressure therapist basically looks at the state of *Qi* (sometimes spelled *Chi* or, in Japanese, *Ki*) and the relationship of Yin and Yang in the body. This is done by enquiring about the nature of the complaint and asking the specific questions that go with pictures – or, rather, patterns – of imbalance.

The Yin and Yang are seen as two polarities in an energetic relationship, Yang always arising from Yin like vigour and strength resulting from good rest and nourishment. Qi describes the energy that is contained in both polarities; it can easily become depleted and needs recharging regularly. We get Qi from the air we breathe, from the food we eat, from the liquids that enter our bodies and the amount of relaxation via sleep and massage, for instance. Unfortunately we tend in our modern lives not to be fully aware of our body's needs, until worsening physical conditions remind us of the necessity to be nurtured at all levels.

Let's look at two examples of the dynamic relationship between

Yin and Yang and the flow of Qi as well as the appropriate energetic response by the Oriental masseur.

When we are stressed we need to rest and so replace vigorous exertion (Yang) with that of rest and nourishment (Yin). There are acupressure points on the body – found along energy lines or conduits called *meridians* – which stimulate different responses because they have been shown to exert various qualities that address the multitude of needs the body has. So the response by the practitioner in this case would be more Yin-oriented: softer work, scattering energy, long strokes. The practitioner would thus seek to disperse energy from the head downwards and outwards by massaging the set of points which include the nourishing and relaxing qualities of Yin.

Suppose a person came into the practice with a flu that had been contracted only a day or two before, with a headache and raised temperature, the pulse beating like a drum and tense muscles around the top of the body. In this case the pathogenic influence has attacked the defences of the body (Wei-Qi) which are vigorously opposing the invading factor (evil-Qi). The energy tends to get blocked on the surface of the body (Yang-place), creating stress-like patterns. Here the pattern is a little more complicated and the treatment would be composed of warming and dispelling techniques, employing kneading and vibrating which have a warming and moving effect. Also, blood would be brought to the surface to allow for a better oxygenation of tissues leading to increased powers of the immune system over the pathogens. A set of points from the Lung-meridian would be chosen as principal points in order to relax the surface and dispel 'wind-cold'.

'Wind' in this context is seen as a general term to denote disharmonious movement that can lead to a disruption of internal functions when attacking from outside. Every changing season has its period of predominating wind – of influences which are potentially harmful to the immune system and to the strength of tendons and ligaments. Little wonder that I as a practitioner see most patients complaining of sciatica, slipped disc problems, frozen shoulder and so forth either in the Spring, which is sometimes called the 'wind season', or in the Autumn when the weather is turning towards Winter and brings lots of stormy and cold damp weather patterns.

CATEGORIES OF MASSAGE

Chinese massage has enjoyed a very long tradition and is as strong as ever. It is taught at college level and in many other places – for example in monasteries or martial-arts training centres – which is why there are a number of systems and styles in practice today. They roughly fall into two groups. The first can be called general massage (*Pu Tong An Mo*), which employs techniques that largely ease and relax stress and in this fashion rebalance the Yin/Yang equilibrium. Some physicians of antiquity termed this the noblest form of medicine because it simply chases away a problem at a point where it would not have the strength to disrupt one's life – which is often of vital importance when burdened with the responsibility of a family or otherwise. This general relaxation massage moves away toxic acids in the tissue, induces restful sleep and rebalances the endocrine system. All the adrenaline shocks received in moments of anxiety and tension during the normal working day tend to tie up a lot of energy which is lost from the digestive system, for instance, which in turn can lead to ulceration of the stomach and the problems associated with chronic fatigue syndrome. By rebalancing the forcefield between Yin and Yang we experience more radiance and vitality, with a stronger immune system and a better quality of life generally. This is why massage is so immensely popular in China, Japan and India, all countries with a very long and old tradition that includes ancient medicinal therapies.

Conventional medicine is more concerned with understanding exactly whether a disease is either bacterial, viral or fungal, specializing in microbiology and all that follows. The *Nei Jing* describes this attitude as such:

> *When medicinal therapy is initiated only after someone has fallen ill, when there is an attempt to restore order only after unrest has broken out, it is as though someone has waited to dig a well until he is already weak with thirst.*

The second category of massage is what we here understand as 'Acupressure'. It is termed *Dian Xue An Mo* in Chinese, which roughly translates as 'cavity press massage'. The acupoints along the meridians are actually seen as cavities in the energy field of Qiflow in the meridians, and finger technique is used to treat a similar selection of points as are often prescribed in acupuncture. 'Acu' in fact derives from the Greek root 'Acus' meaning needle, which doesn't exactly apply to massage techniques. It just happens to be an error in translation which is probably too late to adjust in our common usage.

Some researchers in the field have equated the Qi-force with bio-electricity, because this can be picked up with very sensitive measuring gadgets. Also, new research suggests treating these acupoints with tiny charges of electricity, because it is at these points where the field resistance of electricity is reduced and therefore 'cavity-pressing techniques' effect therapeutic results.

WHAT TO EXPECT FROM A VISIT TO A THERAPIST

Treatment with acupressure consists of various consultations depending on the severity of the problem presented. When a person comes to see me, we talk over the condition first, then I will have a look at the tongue (to see the strength of the pathogenic factor) and feel the pulse (to 'listen' to the strength of Qi). From here we can proceed to more specialized questions and start refining the picture into a treatment strategy. The treatment will usually last for one hour.

CONDITIONS FOR WHICH IT IS EFFECTIVE

To illustrate the type of problems that can be addressed with acupressure, here is a (by no means comprehensive) list of the most commonly seen ailments:

Common cold
Sleeplessness
Cramps
Headaches
Stiff neck and shoulders
Lumbago
Joint problems
Allergies
Asthma and breathing difficulties
Sciatica
Tendonitis
Carpal tunnel syndrome
Hypertension
Jet-lag
Depleted immune system
Adrenal fatigue
Nervousness
Sluggish circulation
Palpitations
Stomach/liver/kidney/lung and heart problems

QUALIFICATIONS

The Acupressure practitioner has to have studied the same complex theory of Chinese anatomy and physiology, aetiology and pathology as his acupuncture counterpart. This is indispensable to understand clearly the diagnosis and treatment principle, and be familiar with many symptom pictures. This takes a number of years to master.

Register of Traditional Chinese Medicine (RTCM)
19 Trinity Road
London N2 8JJ
Tel. 081–883 8431

Further Reading
Jacqueline Young, *Acupressure for Health* (Thorsons, 1994)
Julian N. Kenyon, *Acupressure Techniques* (Thorsons, 1987)

❧ ACUPUNCTURE ❧

LYNN OSBORNE AND EVE ROGANS

ORIGINS

Chinese medicine comes to us from a long, long history. Five thousand years ago the Taoist tradition (of which Chinese medicine is a part) was an oral tradition only passed on from family to family by stories, poems and myths.

> *All people come to those who keep the one*
> *For there lies happiness and peace*
> *Passers-by may stop for music and good food*
> *But a description of the Tao*
> *seems without substance or flavour.*
> *It cannot be seen, it cannot be heard,*
> *And yet it cannot be exhausted.*

It did not become a written form until 3000 BC when the *Nei Jing* was established. This comprised the 'Su Wen' and the 'Ling Shu', a medical treatise and the spiritual discipline which underlies it respectively.

The development of Acupuncture needles began in 1766–1154 BC (Sheng Dynasty). Doctors began to use stone probes to adjust the flow of energy in the body and help their patients maintain harmony in the body, mind and spirit. Acupuncture is one way of establishing this harmony within the Taoist tradition. It is known as one of the strands of the eight brocades; the other seven are herbal therapy, dietary therapy, thermogesis (heat treatments), Taoist massage, Acupuncture, Tai Qi and Qigong.

Since 3000 BC there have been many dynasties in China and much change in Chinese culture. With each dynasty and each culture have come new doctors who have sought to help human suffering and sickness using Taoist techniques. This has left us with a rich diversity of prescriptions and formulae. Spanning the universal ancient works of the Taoists and the modern techniques offered in China today, there is always something in Traditional Chinese Medicine (TCM) for the individual in his or her current need.

PHILOSOPHY

Since this system of medicine began, some things have not greatly changed; these are the laws of nature and the human being's place within these laws.

Chinese medicine does not separate a person's health from his or her position in the universe, spiritual aspirations, emotional world or ability to be independent and self-sufficient. The more we understand ourselves, our connections and our effects upon our world, the more power and strength we can have, and the more fulfilled and loving we can be. We can help ourselves to do this by understanding the underlying philosophy of Chinese medicine.

The nameless is the beginning of heaven and earth
The named is 10,000 things.

The nameless is Chi (Qi), or spark, or energy, that moves in everything and is at the heart of Taoist philosophy. It is part of everything and it organizes itself to become everything. When it becomes water it is wet and flows, when it becomes fire it is hot and rises up, when it is air we breathe it in. It changes in the body and we breathe it out as carbon dioxide. It is all Chi and it changes its form but it is still Chi. Everything is connected by it and when we understand it we can use it positively both within ourselves and our environment. If we are exhausted because Chi is not flowing in the body, we can learn to unblock it, in this case with needles, but diet or exercise or a change in mental attitude can have the same effect.

The Chinese first described Chi as polarizing into Yin and Yang.

> *Under heaven all can see beauty as beauty*
> *Only because there is ugliness*
> *All can know good as good*
> *Only because there is evil*
> *Therefore having and not having arise together.*
> *Difficult and easy complement each other*
> *High and low rest upon each other*
> *Voice and sound harmonize each other*
> *Front and back follow one another.*

Once you describe one thing as bound in time then you must create its opposite or its balance – but these are not static opposites, they are also changing. Day changes into night, Summer into Winter, laughter to sadness, fullness to emptiness. In the body we look at balancing Yin and Yang. When people are Yin-deficient they may be hot, over-active, dry, speak rapidly, not sleep enough and get ravenous. If the Yang is deficient, there may be slowness of movement, lethargy, sleepiness, poor appetite, sogginess and wetness in the body.

It is the role of the practitioner to facilitate change by rebalancing the energy. Where there is too much cold we warm, and where there is too much heat we cool the energy.

After Yin and Yang the Taoists further differentiated everything into five elements, or *Wuxu* ('five moving forces'). These are wood, fire, earth, metal and water. Here we see that in Chinese medical thinking, as in Taoist philosophy, one thing is not separate from another. Chi is bound only by time and space. So, in the human being the Chi makes the human, organizes itself into Yin and Yang aspects and then further branches into wood, fire, earth, metal and water.

It is an important aspect of Chinese medicine to realize that nothing is static. There is always a concept of change and growth; everything is on a continuum. While evaluation is important judgement is suspended, because judgement can cause blocking, whereas evaluation allows the process to continue.

> *The ten thousand things rise and fall without cease*
> *creating yet not possessing*
> *Working yet not taking credit.*
> *Work is done, then forgotten,*
> *Therefore it lasts forever.*

When patients come with an illness it is seen as part of a whole changing dynamic in their lives, something to direct them in terms of their health and destiny, not something that is static or separate from them. This avoids a lot of over-identification with negative aspects of the self and it promotes the patient towards self-responsibility and health. In this way the patient has a direction to aim for and can learn from the symptoms. This helps patients to regain their health and take more control over themselves and the natural world in which they live. This is an important aspect of the return to health: it allows patients to work with, rather than against nature.

HOW IT WORKS

The Five Elements

This section will be an integrated approach to the five elements including positive representational models. Having understood the basic philosophy of Chinese medicine and Yin and Yang and the five elements, we now turn to look at the mechanics of the procedure of acupuncture. Acupuncture seeks to balance these energies in the body by the use of fine needles placed into specific points. Each point has its own function and is placed on a system of meridians or channels.

Diagnosis

This is complex and will be described later in the text, but basically the practitioner is looking for either internal or external causes of disease. These blocks cause Chi not to flow as it should. The external causes are when too much cold, heat, damp, wind or dryness invades the system. This normally occurs because the system is already weak.

The internal causes of dis-ease are the five emotions – an excess of either joy, worry, grief, fear or anger – that has not been resolved. These influences affect the Chi of the body and have to be freed to continue the flow. With external causes of dis-ease it is necessary for patients to look at lifestyle management; with internal, emotional and spiritual management.

WHAT TO EXPECT FROM A VISIT TO A THERAPIST

Now let's look at a visit to the Acupuncturist and how these concepts and techniques are applied in practice.

On your first visit to an Acupuncturist you will be asked in detail about your reasons for coming. Then you will be asked many questions about your health generally, including your emotional health and lifestyle, which you may not think relevant to your present condition but which help to build up a complete picture. This will contribute to your traditional Chinese diagnosis, from which your therapist will be able to decide how to treat you.

After this, the Acupuncturist will take your pulse and ask to see your tongue. The Acupuncturist will place her first three fingers on either wrist in turn to feel the radial artery. Traditional Chinese Medicine (TCM) does not consider the pulse in the way that Western medicine does. In TCM we are feeling the quality of the different pulses under the fingers, rather than just the rate of the heart. Each finger will feel the energy of a particular organ–meridian and how that meridian is functioning in the body. There are 28 different pulse qualities listed, with names such as wiry, slippery, deep floating, choppy, tight and so on. It is important to feel the overall quality of the pulse and therefore Qi in the body, as well as to recognize any organ–meridians that may stand out as being obviously different.

There are several pulse pictures we can refer to – they are similar but vary slightly – and it is important to use different pressures when feeling the pulse: heavier pressure feels the Qi of the Yin organs; lighter, the Yang organs.

The tongue is also a very important diagnostic tool in TCM; sometimes it is even more important than the pulse, as it changes much more slowly and reflects the true inner condition of the person without responding to different situations (such as stress or exercise), as the pulse does. We look at the colour of the tongue body itself and study the lines on it; we also consider the quality, colour and shape of the tongue. A pale tongue will reflect a more Yin, cold condition, while a too-red tongue will show Yang or heat. A normal tongue is light red. The tongue coating is very important, especially in showing the state of the digestive organs. A normal coating is thin and white. A thick, dry and yellow coating shows the presence of phlegm – heat in the body which has consumed the Yin fluids. A thick damp white coating indicates a damp, cold condition inside. There are infinite variations in the tongue and pulse, and diagnosing these variations constitutes the skill of the Acupuncturist.

After the Acupuncturist has asked all these questions, taken your pulse and looked at your tongue, she will make a TCM diagnosis and decide which acupuncture points to needle. You will then undress and lie down on the treatment table. The therapist will insert the needles one by one, and then leave them in for about 20 minutes. You may feel a little prick when some of the needles go in, though you may not feel them at all.

As soon as each needle is inserted you may feel a short-lived sensation, which can be a twinge, shooting, tingling, numbness or a sensation you cannot describe. This is called *Deqi* and it happens when the needle 'grabs' the Qi. It may be somewhat startling but it is a positive response and should be welcomed. It is important to relax and 'breathe through it', for if you tense your muscles it can be more painful. This sensation passes in a moment, after which you relax and lie still for 20 minutes. This is not as difficult as it sounds, for your muscles do relax very soon after the needles are inserted, and may start to feel quite heavy. You may become quite dreamy and often drift off into daydreams or even snooze! Afterwards you may feel a little light-headed and quite relaxed. You should probably have eaten something a little while before acupuncture, though nothing too heavy. It is often a good idea to sit and have a cup of tea afterwards before rushing off too quickly.

HOW IT FITS INTO AN INDIVIDUAL'S LIFESTYLE

Treatment is generally given weekly. As you start to feel better and your symptoms improve, your treatments may then become more spaced out. It is impossible to say how many treatments constitute a course, as each person's state of health is different. However, as Acupuncture affects your energy a little bit at a time, building up gradually until a more permanent change is effected, it *is* important to complete a course of treatment. If you come in with an acute disease, which acupuncture can help quickly, then you may only need a few treatments in quick succession. The first session naturally takes longer, as we go through an extensive personal and medical history. Subsequent sessions last between 30 minutes and an hour.

Your Acupuncturist will also talk about changes you may need to make in your lifestyle that will enable you to feel better and stay generally healthier. Acupuncture can do a great deal, but if you are persistently doing something that is working against your healing, the results will not be sustained. This may include advice on suitable types of exercise, giving up smoking, and changes in diet. All advice within TCM is tailored to you personally, to help your Yin/Yang balance. For instance, if you have a Kidney Qi weakness, you will be asked to keep your lower back warm, to lift carefully, not to have too much sex, and not to get overtired. Much of this is common sense, once you follow the principles of Yin/Yang.

Similarly, most foods are classified as having hot or cold energies, or an infinite variety in between. If your energy is too cold and slow (Yin), you will be asked to avoid dairy produce, ice-cream, watermelon and many cold and raw foods. You don't have the Yang heat to process them properly and they will further clog you up and slow you down. You will instead be advised to eat cooked (not spicy) foods, root vegetables, onions, garlic and ginger (more Yang). All these things put heat into the body and help it to transform your food properly so as to build up your Qi.

HOW IT INTERACTS WITH OTHER THERAPIES

Acupuncture goes very well with several other therapies. It is particularly good with **Traditional Chinese Herbalism**, where the diagnosis is made from the same medical tradition. Often, the herbs will help clear up a long-standing deficiency while the acupuncture can deal with the immediate problem you have come about. Sometimes it can help shift a long-standing phlegm-damp in the digestive system much more quickly than Acupuncture alone.

If you come with a back problem, Acupuncture can help considerably; however, if it does not improve beyond a certain point, we may recommend you see an Osteopath or Chiropractor (**Chiropractic**). Acupuncture and Osteopathy can work very well in tandem and often effect a more complete change than either one alone. **Cranial Osteopathy** is particularly suited to Acupuncture, as the cranial rhythms are very similar to Qi and Cranial Osteopathy is a holistic way of looking at the body.

Other therapies that work with the vital energy may be less compatible with Acupuncture; however, on the whole, most Acupuncturists do not see these therapies as an obstacle to treatment. If you have too many therapies at any one time, though, your Qi may not have time to recover and assimilate any one treatment. Your therapist will advise you on this matter.

CONDITIONS FOR WHICH IT IS EFFECTIVE

The range of conditions that Acupuncture can help is very wide and includes:

Gynaecological problems
Lung problems
Digestive problems, including liver and gallbladder problems
Urogenital disorders
Emotional and stress problems
Sleep disorders
Allergies
Skin disorders

Circulatory problems
Ear, nose and throat (ENT) problems
Nerve disorders – e.g. sciatica, paralysis
Obstetric difficulties
Sexual difficulties
Addictions – smoking, tranquillizers, heroin, alcohol
Infectious diseases – measles, mumps, flu, etc.
Auto-immune disorders – Rheumatoid arthritis, Multiple
    Sclerosis, Myalgic encephalomyelitis (ME).

Many other diseases can be treated – those listed above help give an idea of the wide-ranging scope of Acupuncture.

QUALIFICATIONS

All British Acupuncturists should be members of one of the five different organizations that make up the Council for Acupuncture (CfA). These are the British Acupuncture Association & Register (BAAR), Chung San Acupuncture Society (CSAS), International Register of Oriental Medicine (IROM), Register of Traditional Chinese Medicine (RTCM – see address above, page 77), and the Traditional Acupuncture Society (TAS). A Register of British Acupuncturists is kept at Neal's Yard Therapy Rooms, should you need someone elsewhere in the British Isles.

Being a member of one of these organizations means the completion of a proper course of training, lasting two to four years, and the possession of medical insurance. It means we are properly regulated and agree to abide by the CfA's common standards of ethics and conditions. As part of the EC's common medical regulations, we are working towards registration of all Acupuncturists, so that the profession as a whole can be properly regulated. The CfA is also a member of a larger British body, the

Council for Complementary and Alternative Medicine (CCAM – for address, see page 14). The CCAM has representation in Parliament and is active in the EC policy-formulation for Complementary medicine.

British Acupuncture Association & Register (BAAR)
34 Alderney Street
London SE1 4EU
Tel. 071–834 1012

The Council for Acupuncture
Suite 1
19 Cavendish Square
London W1M 9AD
Tel. 071–409 1440

Further Reading
Paul Marcus, *Thorsons Introductory Guide to Acupuncture* (Thorsons, 1991)
G. T. Lewith and N. Lewith, *Modern Chinese Acupuncture* (Thorsons, 1984)

ACUPUNCTURE
⤾ AND CHILDREN⤿

EVE ROGANS

Acupuncture is eminently suitable for children and often works very quickly where other medicines fail. Many times, three to six treatments are all that are needed to cure a relatively chronic condition. In Traditional Chinese Medicine (TCM) there are differences in emphasis in how we look at children as opposed to adults, and there are certainly differences in treatment.

Inside the womb, children do not have to use their digestive organs, so their digestion is often weak for a while after birth. This means they may find it difficult to digest many foods properly, including those foods through their mother's milk. Unsuitable foods can cause problems around weaning time and even for a couple of years after. 'Unsuitable foods' for babies may include cow's milk, wholefoods, raw foods, spicy foods or additives.

A weak digestion or, as we say in TCM, 'Spleen deficiency' can be the root cause of many ailments including eczema, constipation, abdominal pain, vomiting, diarrhoea, a cough and asthma. Extra stress, such as emotional upset in the parents, teething, infections or immunizations can aggravate the problem. Immunization or infectious diseases can be the cause of what TCM calls 'Lingering Pathogenic Factor' (LPF). This means that the child has not been able to throw off the pathogenic factor (virus or bacteria) introduced into the body via immunization or infection. This can also be the cause of many problems, either physical (e.g. digestive problems, a cough), emotional or behavioural. One of the signs of LPF is swollen glands in the neck.

It is a good idea to ask your children's Acupuncturist for advice on immunizations. If possible, let your child have some treatment before immunization to make sure the eliminative functions are working properly, and shortly afterwards, to enable the child to throw off the effects more easily.

Children also have a tendency to get hot or feverish more readily than adults, and for this heat to deplete their Yin much more quickly. Their illnesses may rapidly become serious; prompt Acupuncture treatment, possibly once a day for two or three days, can easily bring a child back to health. Hot diseases are often treated with antibiotics these days, and while these can reduce infection, they do leave 'damp phlegm' in the body which may itself cause problems. Even after antibiotics, one or two treatments to allow this phlegm to disperse is a good idea. Acupuncture helps keep a child well and in a better state of health and energy than may have been the case before.

Emotional problems can affect children as well as adults. These can range from testing their will in the 'terrible twos' to responding to pressure at school from the age of seven upwards. Babies and children easily reflect the anxiety or irritation of their parents. Acupuncture can help their Qi find its proper path again.

WHAT TO EXPECT FROM A VISIT TO A THERAPIST

Treatment of children is much simpler than adults, with fewer points. The needles are generally not left in, but once inserted, *Deqi* is obtained and they are immediately removed. With some older children, they may be left in for between five and 10 minutes. Acupuncturists use particularly fine small needles with a special technique for children. Patients do not usually feel the needles go in but they might feel it when they 'catch' (get *Deqi*). Children often look startled when this happens and sometimes cry. Because the pain is very short-lived, however, they are easily distracted and get over it quickly.

CONDITIONS FOR WHICH IT IS EFFECTIVE

Children usually improve much more quickly than adults with Acupuncture and the results can be remarkable. It cannot be overemphasized how beneficial Acupuncture can be to their present and future health. Among the childhood diseases Acupuncture can treat are:

Infectious diseases – flu, mumps, measles, whooping cough
Cough – acute or chronic
Pneumonia, bronchitis
Asthma
Tonsillitis
Digestive disorders – irregular bowels, failure to thrive, abdominal pain, vomiting, diarrhoea
Oral thrush and mouth ulcers
Convulsions and epilepsy
Bedwetting
Mental retardation and learning disabilities
Teething
Hyperactivity
Eczema and rashes
Short sight and squint
Otitis media (middle ear infection)
Lymph-gland swelling.

❧ ALEXANDER TECHNIQUE ❧

MAX RUTHERFORD

ORIGINS

Frederick Matthias Alexander (F. M. for short) was born in Tasmania in 1869. As a young man he became an actor specializing in Shakespearean monologues. He was in his early twenties and already launched on a promising career when he began to be troubled by a hoarseness of the throat towards the end of each performance. Doctors informed him that his vocal cords had become inflamed, but subsequent medical treatment proved ineffective.

The problem grew worse as time went by, yet during ordinary speaking would not occur. F. M. reasoned that since it was only in the theatre that the problem revealed itself it must be as a result of something that he was doing to himself when he performed and therefore something that could be investigated. This realization led to an extended period of self-observation, with aid of a three-way mirror and a great deal of patience and determination.

What Alexander Discovered

After setting up his mirror Alexander was at first unable to notice anything out of the ordinary, but after a while a pattern emerged.

> *I was particularly struck by three things that I saw myself doing. I saw that as soon as I started to recite, I tended to pull back my head, depress the larynx, and suck in breath through the mouth in such a way as to produce a gasping sound.*

As F. M. became more observant he began to notice the same pattern, but to a lesser degree, in ordinary speaking and a range of other activities. He further noticed that in pulling his head 'back and down', his torso decreased in overall length and width because he arched his back and thrust his chest out while his legs became stiff with tension. He concluded that he was dealing with a total pattern of misuse that involved his entire body and not just one single area. Thus came the important realization that in treating any *specific* area of the body one must also consider the *whole*, otherwise problems are likely to recur again and again.

PHILOSOPHY

Many people, these days, have heard of the Alexander Technique but there is often great confusion as to what it is all about. The author Aldous Huxley, who had lessons with Alexander himself in the 1920s, said that explaining the technique was like trying to describe the colour red to a blind man. One can use a thousand words but none can replace the actual sensations of perception (what you see you see — what you feel you feel).

Words to explain the Alexander Technique are similarly inadequate because awareness of the body is at the level of sensation. Just as vision is one of the original five senses, awareness of the body is now understood to be the sixth, or kinaesthetic, sense. The kinaesthetic sense receives information from sensory nerve endings located in bone and muscle tissue and combines this with information from other sources to inform us of our position in space, of how each part is arranged in relation to all others and the level of tension in the muscles at any given time.

The Alexander Technique aims to increase conscious awareness and understanding of this kinaesthetic sense and thereby improve our sense of ourselves. It is a process of learning similar to that which takes place with the study of music and art or the appreciation of a fine wine. These skills are acquired through exposure to sensory stimulation of a specific kind, on a regular basis; the Alexander Technique operates in much the same way. The teacher helps the pupil to become aware of habitual patterns of movement which interfere with balance and co-ordination, thereby creating unnecessary tension. By subtle manipulation the teacher is then able to facilitate the correction of these habits by giving the pupil an experience of moving in a better way. The whole process has as much to do with how we think as what we do, and with increasing exposure to the technique it becomes clear, from *experience*, that mind and body are one. The critical factor in this learning, however, is the experience and not the words used to describe it. The colour red is something that the blind can only guess at.

HOW IT WORKS

Since Alexander's harmful use involved his entire body, he had to find out where to begin focusing his corrective effort – with his faulty breathing, his misuse of the larynx or with the balance of the head? As he wrote in his book *The Use of the Self*, 'I found myself in a maze.' The route to the centre of the maze was fraught with difficulties but he finally discovered that the total pattern was initiated from the head down and involved the relationship between head, neck and torso – what he termed *the primary control*. This led to the formulation of the three main aspects of the technique:

1. The importance of the primary control.
2. The use of conscious inhibition as an important first step.
3. The use of directed awareness for the control of movement.

The Primary Control

Alexander found his voice failing whenever he pulled his head back and down. In correcting this habit (no easy matter) his back would lengthen and widen and his voice improve. How is it possible that the balance of the head can have such a profound effect on the rest of the body? To understand how this works, imagine the spine as a large spring with guy ropes attached (like those around a tent) and a football sitting on the top. If the tension in the guy ropes is increased the spring will become shorter; if the tension is decreased it will become longer.

The human torso works in much the same way, with the spine acting like a spring and the muscles of the spine and torso acting like guy ropes. In this case, the balance of the head on top of the spine determines the degree of tension (or pulling down) in the muscles. Thus pulling the head back tends to shorten the spine, while releasing it forwards-and-up allows the spine to lengthen (please note, forwards in 'forwards-and-up' indicates a rotational movement and *not* sticking the chin out).

One then has to ask the question, 'Why do we habitually pull our heads back and down as we go into movement?' One reason is that the weight of the skull is two-thirds in front of the point of balance, so that in a skeleton without muscles the head would tend to fall forwards onto the chest. The pull of the muscles attaching to the back of the skull should exactly balance this forwards movement, but we tend to overwork those muscles and pull the head back too far.

When Alexander first noticed this tendency in himself he assumed that correction would be an easy matter, but – although he could maintain a better balance as long as he was doing nothing – as soon as he tried to use his voice for speaking the habit would return. The working out of this problem took quite some time and led him to form the concepts of inhibition and direction.

Conscious Inhibition and Direction

The main reason why Alexander found it so difficult to overcome his habitual preparation for the use of his voice was that any *new* balance of the head always felt 'wrong' to him and so he would automatically slip back into his old habit at the actual moment of speaking. This is how he described the problem:

> *I was suffering from a delusion that is practically universal, the delusion that because we are able to do what we 'will to do' in acts that are habitual and involve familiar sensory experiences, we shall be equally successful in doing what we 'will to do' in acts which are contrary to our habit and therefore involve sensory experiences that are unfamiliar.*

In other words, as long as we continue to use ourselves as we have done in the past we can manage quite well, but as soon as we try to make some small change we experience all kinds of problems. To avoid the unfamiliar feelings which result from trying something new, we tend to revert back to our old, familiar habits, *even when we know them to be harmful or wrong.* Most people will have had some experience of this, for instance when crossing the road in a foreign country, correcting a dance step which turns out to be wrong or making a change of stroke in tennis or golf.

Thus, when learning something new we cannot trust our *feelings* to tell us what is right or what is wrong, because what is familiar and habitual will always feel right while what is new and unfamiliar will always feel wrong. In order to make a change we must therefore make the decision to go against our feelings for the moment and do what we *rationally* know to be right – e.g., when a Briton abroad crosses the road, his instinct tells him to look to the right but he chooses to *override* these feelings and look in the opposite direction because his intelligence tells him to expect traffic from the left. In order to correct bad habits we must therefore rely on some kind of objective feedback. A tennis player will turn to her coach, a musician to a trusted teacher. Alexander learned with the aid of mirrors, and then used his hands to teach others.

What to Expect from Your First Lesson

A typical lesson with a qualified teacher will involve two parts. In the first the pupil, who remains fully clothed throughout, will be asked to lie on a therapeutic couch, face up, in what is known as the *semi-supine* position. This is the most restful position for the spine and involves lying with the head supported on a small pile of books while the knees are balanced in an upright position with feet flat on the couch. Once settled in this position the pupil will be asked to consciously let go while the teacher works to release some of the held-in tension. At times, the teacher will take hold of an arm or a leg and move it around as the pupil works to inhibit any response to the movement which is taking place. In this way the pupil begins to learn the true meaning of inhibition and gets a sense of what it means to move with only the minimum of tension.

During the course of a lesson a teacher can provide the necessary feedback and help us to become aware of how we are going wrong, due to bad habits acquired over a period of years, then give us an experience of moving in new ways which will encourage release (lengthening and widening) rather than a contraction (shortening and narrowing) into movement. In order to facilitate such changes the pupil must make a conscious effort to inhibit the old habits and open up to the possibility of moving in a new way. This simply means learning to keep oneself quiet and free from any unnecessary tension. A bit like wiping the blackboard clean before trying to write something new, you cannot move in a new way if you are still trying, at the same time, to move in the old way. Once you have learned, with the help of the teacher, to inhibit the tendency to contract into movement you must then learn how to direct attention in such a way as to maintain the lengthening for yourself in activity both during and after the lesson.

In all this, the most important factor is learning that *such lengthening is never achieved through 'doing'*. Rather it comes about through the release of habitual tension. Many people think they understand what it means to 'lengthen the spine' but this usually involves tensing up in an effort to make themselves taller. True lengthening can only be achieved through the release of that which pulls us down. Understanding the technique through the written word is, as mentioned above, an impossible task but I hope I have at least inspired you to investigate further.

FOR WHOM IS THE TECHNIQUE INTENDED?

Almost anyone can benefit from lessons in the technique, although some will naturally benefit more than others. Pupils range from those suffering from chronic aches and pains to athletes and performing artists or those under stress who are looking for a way to relax and continue working at one and the same time.

Although the technique has been known, in some cases, to overcome the need for invasive surgery it is important to understand that Alexander teachers are not qualified in medical diagnosis and will always insist on a patient visiting a medical doctor or osteopath in cases where acute pain is presented. The technique is completely harmless and manipulation is gentle throughout, but delays in the treatment of serious pathology must always be avoided wherever possible.

How it Fits into an Individual's Lifestyle

The number of lessons required varies from person to person, but it is best to think in terms of a minimum of 20 lessons spaced over a period of three or four months. This may seem like a lot, but when one considers the time taken to learn to drive, ride a horse or play the piano it can be seen in perspective.

If you are unsure about whether to take lessons the best thing to do is phone a teacher and ask. The technique is no miracle cure and involves a certain amount of commitment on the part of both pupil and teacher, but I believe it is well worth the effort for anyone interested in overcoming some of those old habits which prevent us from moving with ease and from expressing ourselves from the heart.

Qualifications

The majority of Alexander Teachers working in Britain are members of the Society of Teachers of the Alexander Technique (STAT). To qualify as a member of STAT, teachers will have passed through a three-year (1600 hours minimum) full-time course at one of a number of training centres around the UK.

Society of Teachers of the Alexander Technique (STAT)
20 London House
266 Fulham Road
London SW10 9EL
Tel. 071–352 0828

Further Reading
Jonathan Drake, *Thorsons Introductory Guide to the Alexander Technique* (Thorsons, 1993)

❧ APPLIED KINESIOLOGY ❧

SHIRLEY TOPOLSKI

ORIGINS

The word 'applied' translates as 'to put to practical use' and the word 'Kinesiology' derives from the Greek 'the study of motion'. In this case the meaning is the relationship between the muscles and the lymphatic and vascular systems to the mechanics of bodily motion.

Applied Kinesiology was originated in the US in 1964 by a chiropractor, Dr George Goodheart, who began research while conducting a busy Chiropractic Clinic. Increasingly he encountered difficulties in maintaining relief after successful Chiropractic treatments and was drawn to investigate causes other than purely mechanical damage to the skeletal structure, such as the condition and function of the internal organs. This in turn led him to explore and test the groups of muscles surrounding the problem vertebrae, often finding painful nodules which would respond to massage and disperse. On retesting these muscles, Dr Goodheart would find that they had strengthened, affording general relief. This led into a technique of muscle therapy called 'Origin and Insertion' which was the forerunner of Applied Kinesiology.

In those early days of experimentation other Chiropractors began studying these techniques and started correlating the findings between Applied Kinesiology and X-rays, using the former as an aid in locating the precise area of discomfort along the spine.

This in turn led Dr Goodheart to research the relationship between muscle weakness and other physical, mental and emotional conditions, discovering that he had found a valuable tool with which to approach his patients in a more truly holistic way. It is from these humble origins that Applied Kinesiology developed into a diagnostic art, drawing many diverse practitioners into the field of research.

HOW IT WORKS

In all there are 42 muscle tests related to different organs and bodily systems. These can be broken down into the 14 indicator muscles, used primarily in assessing a patient. The other groups of muscles can be used for further in-depth investigations, each muscle being meticulously tested with a light but firm pressure lasting two to three seconds. The preferred method of testing is with the patient lying comfortably horizontal on a treatment couch. The patient is made aware that it is not a contest of strength and is asked to breathe normally, exhaling at the moment of testing. The Kinesiologist is looking to find whether the muscle being tested will lock into place for the duration of the test, or for the extent to which the muscle weakens, begins shaking, or feels excessively heavy to maintain by the patient. In general, muscle testing is pain-free and relaxing. Some shoulder, arm, leg and pelvic problems will necessitate the Kinesiologist approaching the patient with a skill and delicacy of pressure, or where possible using a surrogate testee, as in the case of patients who are young children or who have Parkinson's Disease or Multiple Sclerosis. A surrogate testee is a healthy individual whose unimpaired electromagnetic field can be utilized by the practitioner. By the patient touching the surrogate's head or shoulder, there is a transference of energies through to the surrogate which can then be tested by the practitioner. Using Applied Kinesiology in this way, it is a system of evaluating the whole person, not just as a diagnosis of disease.

What to Expect from a Visit to a Kinesiologist

There are five bodily systems to be considered when muscle testing:

1. The nervous system
2. The lymphatic system
3. The vascular system
4. The cerebro-spinal system
5. The acupuncture-meridian system.

To the Kinesiologist the body functions as an integrated whole and is tested as such by approaching the patient with all five systems in mind. The patient can expect a session of Applied Kinesiology to last between 20 minutes and one hour, commencing with the patient's case history notes. There follows muscle testing and re-balancing muscle weaknesses, either by working on the origin and insertion of the muscles by massaging the invariably sore neurolymphatic points located on the body, or by gently holding the neurovascular points located on the head, or stimulating or sedating the meridians by holding the Acupressure points, or by using a muscle test to pinpoint nutritional deficiencies.

Conditions for Which Kinesiology is Effective

A sluggish circulatory or lymphatic system will benefit enormously from these techniques, as indeed will blocked sinuses, neck and back problems, headaches, unrelated pain, general malaise, digestive disorders, irritable bowel problems, candida, adrenal exhaustion, ME (Myalgic Encephalomyelitis) as well as emotional debility, fears and phobias. An added advantage of Kinesiology is that muscle testing can uncover latent food allergies and vitamin and mineral deficiencies. By placing the suspected food in the mouth or by holding it against the jaw the Kinesiologist can perceive a change in the muscle test. Applied Kinesiology works directly on our electromagnetic field: as our bodies react, the Kinesiologist can take a reading. The muscles will weaken if the patient is sensitive to a food, or will strengthen if the patient is in more need of it. In this way it is possible to investigate the patient's whole diet in a couple of sessions. The findings of such investigation will greatly enhance the progress toward optimum health and in turn is complementary with many other forms of therapy such as **Acupuncture**, **Aromatherapy**, **Chiropractic**, **Homeopathy**, **Osteopathy** and **Herbal Medicine**, to name but a few.

QUALIFICATIONS

Therapists in the UK holding the title 'Graduate of the Academy of Systematic Kinesiology' or 'Balanced Health Instructor of the Academy of Systematic Kinesiology' are recognized Applied Kinesiology practitioners.

A register of Practitioners is available from:

Mr B. Butler
39 Browns Road
Surbiton
Surrey KT5 8ST
Tel. 081–399 3215

Further Reading
Anthea Courtenay and Maggie La Tourelle, *Thorsons Introductory Guide to Kinesiology* (Thorsons, 1992)

❧ Aromatherapy ❧

LOTTE ROSE

Origins

Aromatic plants and infused oils were used extensively by the ancients. The Egyptians, Greeks and Romans used aromatic plant material steeped in vegetable base oils or fats. The essence produced by the aromatic plants dissolved in the base were used for external applications: massage, ointments, etc.

Aromatherapy today uses distilled oils from aromatic plants which are known as essential oils. This distillation process was discovered in the Arab world (attributed to Avicenna) in the 10th century. The essential oils became known as 'The Perfumes of Arabia' and were brought back to Europe by the Crusading knights. Stills were also brought back and local aromatic plants distilled. Essential oils have formed a part of herbal medicine since that time. Essential oils can also be extracted by pressing (as in citrus rinds) and, for flower oils, by a method known as enfleurage or by solvent extraction. The best quality oils are those extracted from the fresh plant material reared without agricultural chemicals to ensure that no residues are present in the essential oil.

Aromatherapy as we know it today has its roots in these earliest methods and has been developed as a body therapy during this century. Essential oils have had a continuous use in cosmetics and perfumes and have been scientifically investigated and their properties verified. For instance, Dr Jean Valnet (a French army surgeon) documented his use of essential oils in treating war wounds during the French war in Vietnam. He also used essential oils with other patients, particularly psychiatric patients, in his civilian practice.

Aromatherapy Today

Today Aromatherapy is used increasingly in hospitals and hospices in the UK as a recognized alternative to chemical sedatives, to aid sleep and to ease patients' discomfort.

Essential oils are highly concentrated substances, their therapeutic properties deriving from the aromatic plant. They have a marked effect both on the body and on the state of mind and spirit.

Aromatherapy treatment uses essential oils to heal the whole person. The essential oils will affect the physical body through their anti-infectious, anti-spasmodic, analgesic and other qualities. There will also be an action on the state of mind. This action comes primarily through the sense of smell. There is a strong link via the limbic area of the brain between the sense of smell and many of our deepest 'survival' functions, such as appetite, sleep patterns, etc. The link between smell and memory is a crucial one in Aromatherapy. When oils are used at home, following treatment, the aroma of the oils will stir the memory of that treatment within the body/mind to continue the healing process. The action of essential oils in Aromatherapy can be seen as the oil that keeps the subtle connective mechanism between body, mind and spirit running smoothly.

WHAT TO EXPECT FROM A VISIT TO A THERAPIST

On the first visit to an Aromatherapist a detailed case history will be taken. This is to enable the Aromatherapist to be aware of any possible contra-indications to certain oils, and to gain an in-depth understanding of the client's needs before choosing the specific essential oils for treatment. Treatments vary depending on the needs of the client, from a massage to ease aches and pains and to relax, to a series of treatments that work on a deeper level to change chronic patterns. For these, essential oils would also need to be used by the client every day in treatments at home. For instance, chronic or recurring pain (such as sinusitis) would be treated with general and specific face massage, inhalations with essential oils, baths and deep relaxation techniques, with any necessary changes in diet and perhaps some simple exercise routines.

The skill of the Aromatherapist lies in choosing the essential oils or blend of oils which suit the physical and emotional needs and character of the client at that particular time. Since each individual is unique, the Aromatherapist will not necessarily use the same oils for people with the same symptoms but will blend the essential oils to suit each individual as a unique whole. This means taking into account all aspects of that person: lifestyle, state of mind, habits – as well as physical symptoms to treat the underlying causes of these symptoms.

The Aromatherapist is trained to know the properties of the essential oils, their uses and contra-indications and their impact on the more subtle, emotional and spiritual aspects of any person. Combined with a thorough knowledge of the physical action of essential oils, there is an intuitive level of understanding brought to bear on selecting the right blend of oils and type of treatment.

TYPES OF TREATMENT

The principal treatment in Aromatherapy is massage. A few drops of the essential oils are diluted in a suitable vegetable oil base generally diluted from 0.5 to 3 per cent. Treatment may be a full body massage or may concentrate on specific areas. The type of massage will be geared to the individual and generally will seek to induce deep relaxation. The essential oils are absorbed through the skin so that a small amount of the active molecules of the essential oils will circulate through the system. Some essential oils have a specific affinity with organs or systems in the body; others possess a more general action, for example toning, stimulating, regulating or calming. Frequently the action of essential oils in the body is that of a catalyst, working with the body's own healing systems to create harmony and fight infection, etc.

CONDITIONS FOR WHICH AROMATHERAPY IS EFFECTIVE

Aromatherapy can treat many conditions and is particularly effective for those conditions where stress is an element. Stress has an effect on both the physical and mental planes and Aromatherapy is ideal as a treatment because essential oils themselves have an effect on both mind and body. Many chronic conditions can be helped by Aromatherapy treatment, such as those of the skin or respiratory system in particular, or chronic recurring pain (such as in back pain, sinusitis or headaches). Treatment would always include some use of essential oils at home and some relaxation exercises, as well as suggested changes in lifestyle and diet if necessary.

Aromatherapy treatment is gentle, nurturing and smells wonderful, but it can produce profound changes in the body/mind system.

HOW IT INTERACTS WITH OTHER THERAPIES

Aromatherapy treatment combines well with other treatments such as Osteopathy, because the action of Aromatherapy massage in easing muscle spasm will assist the effectiveness of any bone manipulation and often will reduce the number of manipulations or adjustments required. Some Aromatherapists use **Reflexology** or **Applied Kinesiology** as part of their treatment, and Aromatherapy lends itself well to many forms of healing and energy work.

LYMPHATIC DRAINAGE MASSAGE

How it Works

Lymphatic Drainage Massage is a massage technique which, as the name suggests, works specifically on the lymphatic system. Essential oils are combined with the massage technique to stimulate the lymphatic flow and clear the system of toxins.

The lymphatic system carries fluid round the body in a network of branching vessels. This fluid carries nutrients (particularly fat-soluble nutrients) to the tissues and carries away fluid and toxins from the cells. The lymphatic system also plays a part in combating and preventing infection by carrying the body's infection-fighting 'equipment' round the body. There is a link to the blood circulation through the lymphatic system via the capillaries, where the tiny vessels of the lymphatic system exchange fluid with the equally small blood capillaries. The larger lymphatic vessels connect to the bloodstream underneath the collarbone into the subclavian veins.

The lymphatic system also has collecting points, or nodes, which can be felt as swollen glands under the jaw in infections such as colds or flu. Other nodes are situated in the groin and the armpits. There are larger ducts into which the tiny tubes of the lymphatic system drain in the abdomen and around the heart. In the larger lymphatic ducts the lymph fluid is filtered by lymphatic glands.

Bacteria and other foreign bodies are collected and lymphocytes produced which help the body fight infection by surrounding and neutralizing invaders. The lymphatic system, unlike the blood circulatory system, does not have a central pump and depends on compression from surrounding muscles and general activity of the body to move the lymph around the body.

Conditions for Which it is Effective

The efficiency of the lymphatic flow is affected by lack of exercise, sedentary work or prolonged standing. Lymphatic Drainage Massage, therefore, is used in Aromatherapy to stimulate and cleanse the system and consists of a series of treatments, generally twice a week over a period of weeks. Aromatic baths to help relax and clear toxins and body oils are used to introduce a small amount of essential oil into the body daily.

Lymphatic Drainage is very effective in helping boost the immune system, for instance when the body is prone to recurring infections, or when recovering from a bout of illness. The twice-weekly Lymphatic Drainage Massage and home treatments would be combined with any changes in diet as necessary and an increase in exercise in tandem with deep relaxation exercises to balance mind and body and decrease stress levels.

Lymphatic Drainage Massage is very helpful in easing fluid retention in the body and is used extensively in treating the fatty fluid deposits of cellulite. Cellulite treatment is a long-term treatment spanning three months or more. During the first four to six weeks, twice-weekly massage treatments are necessary. These are combined with daily dry skin-brushing, aromatic baths and self-massage at home. A detoxifying diet is also recommended (to suit the individual's needs and lifestyle) along with a programme of exercise and de-stressing techniques.

As the treatment progresses the frequency of the massages can be reduced but the programme of diet and exercise, baths, etc. will continue. Essential oils are chosen to suit the individual and changed at about three- to four-weekly intervals. The whole person will be treated and essential oils for the emotional and mental state will always be included along with deep relaxation and de-stressing techniques which are integral to the treatment.

Qualifications

An Aromatherapist may hold a qualification as an Associate of Tisserand Aromatherapists (ATA) or a Tisserand Diploma in Holistic Aromatherapy. He or she may belong to the International Society of Practising Aromatherapists (ISPA) or International Federation of Aromatherapists (IFA).

> International Federation of Aromatherapists
> Department of Continuing Education
> Royal Masonic Hospital
> Ravenscourt Park
> London W6 0TN

Further Reading
Julia Lawless, *The Encyclopaedia of Essential Oils* (Element 1992)
Shirley Price, *Practical Aromatherapy* (Thorsons, 1987)
—, *Shirley Price's Aromatherapy Book* (Thorsons, 1993)
Christine Wildwood, *Holistic Aromatherapy* (Thorsons, 1992)

⮞ AUTOGENIC THERAPY ⮜

NIDA MOHYLNYCKY INGHAM

Autogenic Therapy (or 'Autogenics') consists of a number of related methods for assisting the body's self-regulatory processes. It is concerned with achieving mental and physical harmony. Autogenics is not performed on the individual by the therapist but is something which the individual is taught by the therapist to use for him- or herself.

The word 'Autogenics' means 'self-generating' and reflects the fact that Autogenics is not imposed on the individual but rather assists his or her physical and psychological processes. Autogenics has no religious or cultural overtones.

ORIGINS

Autogenic Training originated from research on sleep and hypnosis carried out at the end of the 19th century which showed that some people who had been hypnotized were able to put themselves into a hypnotic-type state with marked recuperative effects. This was taken up in the 1920s by Dr J. H. Schultz, a German doctor interested in finding a therapeutic approach free from the unfavourable aspects of hypnotherapy, such as the dependence of the individual on the therapist. Dr Schultz found that those entering the hypnotic-type state experienced heaviness in the limbs and warmth throughout the body, and that people taught to imagine they were experiencing these feelings with a passive and casual attitude were able to go into the recuperative state of 'passive concentration' now used in Autogenics.

Autogenic theory was developed from these findings by Dr Schultz and by Dr W. Luthe. Largely as a result of Dr Luthe's work, it is now based on a substantial body of scientific research.

PHILOSOPHY

Autogenics is based on the concept that the mind and the body are a unit and that nature has provided homeostatic mechanisms to regulate both relatively simple biological functions (e.g. body temperature and heart rate) and more complicated matters of a psychological nature. Undue stress has an adverse effect on these mechanisms.

According to Autogenic theory, each individual is endowed with a certain genetic potential – 'The Authentic Self' – and healthy development requires a level of pressure which is compatible with this. It is stressful both for a person not to achieve his or her Authentic Self or to be pushed beyond it. Any factors which interfere with the individual achieving the Authentic Self results in the lowering of his or her inner harmony and capacity to adapt. At the psychological level this may mean increased insecurity, tension, anxiety, depression, lowering of motivation and failure to self-actualize. At the organismic level it results in greater tendency to illness. This can occur at any time from conception and constitutes a long-term source of stress.

Autogenic theory assumes that when a person is exposed to excessive disturbing stimulation the brain uses normal biological processes to reduce the upsetting consequences. It assumes that the client's own system knows best how certain functional disturbances came about and how to reduce their effects. Although these processes occur naturally (e.g. during sleep) they tend to be inhibited. Regular practice of Autogenics facilitates and supports these natural processes by altering the brain-wave patterns to a mainly alpha (awake, alert but blank and peaceful) and theta (half-asleep or dreaming) state, by moving the autonomic nervous system from a high arousal (sympathetic-dominated) state to a relaxed, recuperative (parasympathetic-dominated) one and by producing a balancing between the left (analytical, logical) and right (creative, intuitive) sides of the brain.

When learning Autogenics, and particularly in the early stages, clients may experience phenomena known as 'autogenic discharges'. These are discharges by the brain of accumulated disturbing material. When areas of the brain become overloaded with such material, the brain discharges it through its own self-regulatory processes. Autogenics assists these. In the early stages of learning Autogenics it is possible for discharges (e.g. muscular twitches) to occur when practising the exercises. This process is very healthy in that it is freeing the brain of unwanted material, but because of it Autogenics should be learned with a properly qualified therapist who will adapt the process to suit each individual.

CONDITIONS FOR WHICH IT CAN BE EFFECTIVE

Autogenics is especially suited for managing stress and preventing or helping stress-related conditions such as insomnia, anxiety, depression, migraine, hypertension, asthma, gastro-intestinal disorders, skin complaints, arthritis, stuttering, blushing, obesity and alcohol dependence. It helps with illnesses of the immune system such as ME and HIV/AIDS and it helps to cope with stressful situations (e.g. public speaking). Autogenics improves intellectual and creative performance and promotes psychological balance and personal development. It can also help to prepare a woman for pregnancy and childbirth.

Generally, Autogenics can be practised by anyone over five years old. However, there are certain people for whom it is not suited including those with diabetes or epilepsy whose condition is in any way unstable, persons suffering from narcolepsy or acute psychosis and persons taking hard or soft drugs.

There are a number of different forms of Autogenic Therapy. The basic form, which most people find sufficient for their needs, is Autogenic Training. Having learned this, the client can go on to the others: Autogenic Meditation/Advanced Autogenics, Autogenic Neutralization and Creativity Mobilization Technique.

Autogenic Training involves the performance of certain simple mental exercises with a casual and passive attitude (the state of 'passive concentration' referred to earlier) in one of three relaxed postures. The main exercises are:

A. The six standard exercises: verbal formulae focusing on heaviness, warmth and coolness in certain parts of the body, on heart-beat, breathing and a feeling of peace. These can be practised virtually anywhere or at any time.

B. The intentional exercises, which are performed by the client when alone and not overheard. They involve setting in motion the release of emotions or natural reactions and include using unco-ordinated physical movements, crying, 'nonsense noises' and the uninhibited release of aggression and anxiety. Before learning the aggression and anxiety intentionals, clients are encouraged to make a list of the situations which make them angry or anxious, thus helping them to become more aware of those situations and to develop strategies to help deal with them.

C. Personal formulae, which are composed by the client to meet particular personal needs (e.g. lack of confidence, inability to form relationships, desire to stop smoking) and which are psychologically oriented.

D. Two short exercises which are practised out of the Autogenic state and which can be used during stressful situations such as interviews.

How it Fits into an Individual's Lifestyle

Autogenic Training is learned, either in small groups or on an individual basis, in nine weekly sessions with a final session after two months. Generally, individual sessions last an hour and group sessions one and a half hours. Between the weekly sessions the client is required to undertake regular daily practice (a practice session lasting 10 to 15 minutes) and to keep a training diary of his or her practice and experiences during it. Learning Autogenic Training therefore requires motivation.

What to Expect from a Visit to a Therapist

Prior to starting Autogenics a person is required to complete a health questionnaire and to attend a preliminary session. This procedure allows the therapist to assess the client physically and psychologically to check whether Autogenic Training is suitable and to tailor an appropriate course (which may need modification later in the light of progress). In addition the session enables the therapist to enquire why the client wishes to learn Autogenics, to explain what is involved, and to assess motivation. It also gives the client an opportunity to raise points and decide whether he or she wishes to proceed.

If the client proceeds, each session will start with the client and therapist reviewing the past week's practice with particular reference to the training diary. The therapist then teaches the week's exercise and the client practises this under supervision. Beneficial effects will often start to be felt after a few sessions. Once the client has learned Autogenic Training he or she continues to practise it once or twice a day. The beneficial effects accumulate with regular practice.

HOW IT INTERACTS WITH OTHER THERAPIES

Autogenics can be used with any other natural therapy except Hypnosis, which has an adverse effect on the Autogenic state.

FURTHER DEVELOPMENT

Autogenic Meditation/Advanced Autogenics can be learned either individually or in groups by those who are experienced in Autogenics and who do not experience Autogenic discharges. It is learned in seven sessions, each of which involves concentrating on a specific subject in the Autogenic state. The subjects, which are worked through in a structured way, include the spontaneous experience of colours generally, selected colours, the visualization of specific objects (e.g. childhood home), abstract concepts (e.g. love, creativity), states of feeling (looking at the sunset), other persons and answers from the unconscious. Autogenic meditation is used not only for personal development but to help certain disorders (e.g. insomnia).

Autogenic Neutralization is a form of therapy which is undertaken on an individual basis. It may be used to deal with Autogenic discharges which Autogenic Training alone has not dealt with, and for deep-rooted problems. Autogenic Neutralization takes two forms: abreaction and verbalization. Abreaction involves the client going into the Autogenic state and describing everything experienced, e.g. thoughts, emotions, body sensations. The client discusses these experiences with the therapist at the end of the session. The session is tape-recorded and the client afterwards makes a transcript, reads it and adds a commentary. He or she then discusses the experience and commentary with the therapist at the next session. Once the client is sufficiently competent he or she carries on sessions unsupervised at home, discussing them afterwards with the therapist. Autogenic verbalization is similar except the client focuses on a pre-selected topic, e.g. aggression, anxiety or obsessive material.

Creativity Mobilization Technique (CMT) involves 'mess painting' on newspaper sheets using eight standard colours. It is learned in six sessions, usually on a group basis. The painter's aim is to enter into a 'no-thought' state while painting. He or she allows any thoughts and emotions to surface spontaneously no matter what their nature and to engage freely in verbal and motor expression, e.g. yelling, crying, punching. Periods of negative emotion should be worked through until they subside. The client displays his or her pictures and acknowledges them as part of him- or herself. Like the other forms of Autogenics, CMT helps develop creativity. It assists the client achieve self-awareness and discover ways of fulfilling potential. CMT has much in common with the intentional exercises in that it is a means of contacting and releasing blocked memories and emotions.

TRAINING AND QUALIFICATIONS

The development of Autogenics and the maintenance of standards are promoted by an international association of practitioners,

ICAT, and by national bodies – in Britain, the British Association of Autogenic Training and Therapy. Persons wishing to train in Britain as Autogenic therapists need a suitable professional qualification e.g. in medicine, psychotherapy, clinical psychology or counselling. Qualified therapists are restricted to teaching Autogenics to clients suitable to their training and experience.

British Association for Autogenic Training and Therapy
Secretary: Mrs Jane Bird
18 Holtsmere Close
Garston
Watford WD2 6NE
Tel. 0923 675501

Further Reading

W. Luthe, *Stress and Self-Regulation: Introduction to the Methods of Autogenic Therapy* (Pointe-Claire, Quebec: International Institute of Stress, 1977)
—, 'Stress and Autogenic Therapy', in H. Selye (ed.), *Selye's Guide to Stress Research*, Vol. 2 (New York: Van Nostrand Reinhold Co., 1980)
J.H. Schultz and W. Luthe, *Autogenic Therapy*, Vol. 1 (New York & London: Grune & Stratton, 1969)

❧ BACH FLOWER REMEDIES ❧

SUE EVANS

If you have ever stood and gazed over a skilfully planted garden ablaze with banks of colour and with the scent of the flowers drifting in the air, you will have experienced the soothing, balancing and at the same time invigorating effect that can be produced by what are known as subtle energies. There is nothing tangible about these forces, yet their effects are undeniable.

Whereas the more material substance of the plant – taken as a herbal powder, tincture or infusion – can bring about balance in the physical body, the more subtle characteristics or essence of the plant affect primarily the mind, emotions and even the spirit. Some of these characteristics we can perceive, such as scent and colour, but others elude the range of our senses. Nevertheless, like light outside the visible spectrum or sound beyond our range of hearing, these subtle energies exist and can have a powerful effect on us.

It is these energies that form the basis of the Bach Flower System. Each plant possesses a unique combination of these subtle energies which comprise its essence and by which it can be recognized, just as the scent of honeysuckle or jasmine is immediately associated in our minds with those particular plants.

Flower Essences, therefore, can be said to consist of the characteristic subtle energy patterns of various plants. Preserved in a liquid form these essences can be used to balance the emotional body and thus affect our physical well-being. We are all familiar with how emotions can have a direct effect on the physical body: imagine the tension we can create in our neck and shoulders when we are irritable or overstretched at work, tension which can lead to a headache or inability to eat or digest our food. Fear and anxiety can bring about feelings of weakness, light perspiration, trembling and palpitations. Clench your jaw with repressed anger and you will feel the tension affecting the musculature of the front of the neck and chest; likewise clench a fist and you will feel the tensions in the arm, shoulder and into the back down to the base of the ribcage, the site of the liver (right side) and the spleen (left side) – no wonder these organs are affected by long-term anger and resentment. On a happier note we have all seen the healthy glow, tireless energy and resistance to infection of someone in love. A system of medicine which can balance these long-term emotions and relieve their physical effects is indeed a powerful tool.

ORIGINS

Dr Edward Bach was born near Birmingham in 1886. He trained as a doctor and was well known and respected for his work linking chronic disease with various bacterial populations present in the gut. He developed a range of vaccines as a result of his work which are still in use today as homoeopathic potencies. During his years of research Dr Bach was made more and more aware that the true origins of physical illness lie in emotional imbalances. Either the physical condition would build up over a period of time due to particular negative emotional states, or it would have a sudden onset triggered by some extreme trauma, accident, bereavement, etc. Today there is more recognition for an emotional basis to illness and doctors are beginning to recognize certain personality types which predispose particular patterns of illness.

Becoming somewhat disillusioned with the medicine of his day, Bach held to his vision of a system of medicine which was simple, effective and available to all, regardless of class or income. In 1930 he left his successful practice and, taking with him a bare minimum of possessions, he travelled to Wales where he lived simply, working on his new system of healing. Dr Bach was very sensitive to the subtle essence of the plants around him; his perceptions were finely tuned beyond our normal range. Walking in the unspoiled countryside of Wales he would focus his mind on a particular emotion – anger, jealousy, possessiveness, lack of self-confidence – and he would search out the plant that seemed to have a strong healing energy to relieve that emotion. In this way he put together his 12 Healers, the basic Essences of his later system of 38 Healing Remedies. In later years he was to fine-tune his knowledge of the remedies in different ways, but initially he began to work with his new-found remedies and noted the sometimes exceptional results he achieved.

Despite his poverty, Bach always used the best materials for preparing his Essences; somehow there was always just enough money to get by and continue his work. Later in his life he went on to found a centre for continued study and research of his system, work which still continues in the same house to this day, following the precepts laid down by its founder; another centre, equally dedicated to Bach's work and principles, has also now been set up.

WHO CAN BENEFIT?

Dr Bach's system of treatment is meant to be available to all – you do not need any particular medical or other qualification to use it as long as you can pinpoint the underlying emotional causes for your complaint. This is often the hardest thing to do for yourself; it is difficult to be sufficiently objective and someone else may be able to perceive connections that escape even a friend or relative with their preconceived conceptions of your character. It is also true that working with the remedies and reading the accounts of other people's experiences with these Essences deepens our familiarity and understanding of the system. For these reasons people will often seek professional help.

WHAT TO EXPECT FROM A VISIT TO A THERAPIST

For proper prescription of the Flower Essences the practitioner must gain as deep an insight into your character and the emotional forces influencing your actions as possible. Sometimes the underlying causes become apparent very early on and may need just a few questions to differentiate between one remedy and another. At other times the consultation may go on for some time, maybe even up to an hour if there is a lack of clarity in the case. If you are consulting a practitioner who uses Bach Flowers together with some other form of therapy, he or she will have probably gleaned sufficient information during the normal consultation time, although you may be surprised by some of the questions!

HOW BACH FLOWER ESSENCES INTERACT WITH OTHER THERAPIES

Bach Flower Essences can be used with almost any form of therapy. It is often the case, where the impact of the long-term emotional imbalance on the physical body has brought about definite physical malfunction, that it is best to combine the Flower Essences with some other form of treatment such as **Herbal Medicine**, **Acupuncture**, **Reflexology**, etc. Where the emotional states are long term the prescribed Flower Essences will also need time to rebalance the system, and a particular combination, or variations on the combination, may have to be taken for several months for its action to be complete. It may be inappropriate to use the Bach Flower system with Homoeopathy since this therapy also focuses strongly on the emotional body and the use of the Flower Essences may cloud the practitioner's ability to assess the action of the remedies. However, even in cases such as this, the use of Rescue Remedy is often allowed.

Rescue Remedy is a particular combination of Flower Essences that Dr Bach discovered to have an effect very much above and beyond the range of the individual remedies in the mix. It is generally advised for use immediately after any form of physical, mental or emotional trauma – the principle being that, if the effects of the trauma are neutralized straight away, they will not build up to create physical imbalance at a later date. It is impossible to stress sufficiently the importance of this concept or to envisage the extent of later physical suffering that has been prevented by timely use of the Rescue Remedy (or the appropriate homoeopathic remedy).

Following trauma, Dr Bach cites the case of administration of the Rescue Remedy to a man brought out from the sea as dead but fully revived by the time he had been carried up the beach. Administration of the remedy can be on the pulse points or on the lips if it is not possible to take it by mouth. On a less dramatic level it can be used after a bump in the car, a fall, an upsetting phone call, before exams, driving tests, dental appointments, etc. to preserve a calm emotional state. Rescue Remedy can also be obtained as a cream and I have seen fingers, severely crushed in a door, heal completely in two days with no pain or bruising with repeated application of this Rescue Cream. If you had nothing else to hand, the Rescue Remedy could surprise you by some of the results it can achieve.

Had Dr Bach lived longer, he would have undoubtedly continued his research and gone on to discover other healing plant essences. Today, especially as we find our world changing at a rapid pace, we need the healing subtle energies of the plant kingdom to maintain our balance. Just as herbalists, homoeopaths and other therapists are continually expanding their *Materia medicas*, so too we find others have continued Bach's work in the field of Flower Essences. New Essences have been discovered, such as the Californian Flower Essences and the Australian Bush Essences, and many researchers in Britain are expanding our knowledge of our own common healing plants. It is important to keep an open mind and accept these new arrivals on the basis of their merits, for they have much to offer in the work of healing.

Bach Flower Centre
Mount Vernon
Sotwell
Wallingford
Oxfordshire OX10 0PZ
Tel. 0491 39489

The Healing Herbs of Dr Bach
PO Box 65
Hereford
HR2 0UW
Tel. 0873 890218
Make and supply the 38 Flower Remedies, and offer courses and training.

USA
Dr Edward Bach Healing Society
644 Merrick Road
Lynbrook, NY 11563
Tel. 516–593–2206

Further Reading

Edward Bach, *Heal Thyself* (Saffron Walden: C. W. Daniel, 1931)

—, *The Twelve Healers* (Saffron Walden: C. W. Daniel, 1933; available from Flower Remedy Programme, PO Box 65, Hereford HR2 0UN)

Julian and Martine Barnard, *The Healing Herbs of Edward Bach* (Bath: Ashgrove Press, 1993)

Phillip M. Chancellor, *Handbook of the Bach Flower Remedies* (Saffron Walden: C. W. Daniel, 1971)

Gurudas, *Flower Essences and Vibrational Healing* (San Rafael, CA: Cassandra Press, 1983)

Mechthild Scheffer, *Bach Flower Therapy* (Thorsons, 1993)

George Vlamis, *Rescue Remedy* (Thorsons, 1994)

Nora Weeks, *The Medical Discoveries of Edward Bach, Physician* (Saffron Walden: C. W. Daniel, 1980)

❧ CHIROPRACTIC ❧

MILO SIEWERT

TERMINOLOGY

Chiropractic – the science, art and philosophy
Chiropractor – the therapist

WHAT IS CHIROPRACTIC?

Chiropractic is a form of manipulation by hand, for the release of nerve interference causing pain and ill health. This form of therapy is centred primarily on the spine but can help with any joint or organ of the body. The word Chiropractic is derived from the Greek words Cheiro (hand) and Praktos (concerned with action), thus 'hand practice' or manipulation.

Within the spine is the main trunk of nerves to the body; any interference with these nerves or pressure on the nerves by misalignment of the spinal segments causes deranged function of muscles, joints and organs creating disease and ill health.

ORIGINS

The art is not new but dates back to the Chinese and Greeks from as early as 2700–1555 BC. The bone-setters of the 18th–19th centuries were well known and accepted as skilled individuals.

Their skills were handed down from father to son or by on-the-job training. The same was done by the medical profession up to the 1900s. The re-establishment of manipulation was by a non-medical anatomist, D. D. Palmer in 1895, the same year that X-rays were discovered by Wilhelm Roentgen of Würzburg, Germany.

PHILOSOPHY

Dr Palmer reasoned that if he found a segment or vertebral bone of the spine out of alignment with the adjoining ones then this would be the cause of nerve interference and pain or dysfunction. Interestingly, his first patient was a janitor in the building in which he worked, who related he had lost his hearing while in a stooped position and at the time had felt a popping in his back between his shoulders. Dr Palmer examined him and found that a bone seemed out of place in his back and manipulated it back into position, which restored his hearing. This was a rather unusual circumstance as in 37 years' practice I have never had such a remarkable result as that of totally restoring hearing. So, had this first treatment failed, Chiropractic could have been set back a number of years. Fortunately for all of us who have benefited from Chiropractic, the theory worked and the janitor's hearing was restored. Therefore Dr Palmer promulgated the philosophy, science and art of Chiropractic.

ACCEPTANCE OF CHIROPRACTIC

The science of Chiropractic which has developed has become the second largest primary health care treatment after orthodox medicine and is the largest drugless healing profession. Today, science has accepted the numerous studies undertaken utilizing Chiropractic procedures, and Chiropractors are in a professional status comparable to that of any other paramedical personnel. Chiropractors are accepted in some hospitals and by numerous health insurance companies.

CONDITIONS FOR WHICH IT IS EFFECTIVE

The major problems treated by Chiropractic are musculo-skeletal. These include low back, mid-back and cervical pains which include sciatica, slipped disc, knee and ankle problems, rheumatism, lumbago, neuralgia, fibrositis, neck tension, whiplash, headaches, sinus, catarrh, hearing trouble, eye strain, sports injuries, etc.

Interestingly enough, many problems in children are the result of bad posture. Often school furniture is badly designed, in that there is little thought given to the height of the children in relation to desk height, which reflects in the students' work and mental attitude. Hyper-activity can result and, therefore, spinal checks should be made by a Chiropractor at regular intervals. Babies often suffer from colic, crying spells and sleeplessness, so very mild techniques are taught to help correct the supple spines in babies and small children. Older people with joint problems such as arthritis, stiffness, neck pains, dizziness, headaches, etc. respond to special light techniques. They are often grateful to find Chiropractic of such benefit, for many have tried other therapies that have been of little value or have resulted in bad side-effects.

Pregnant women can also be helped with the multitude of physical changes that take place during the period up to delivery. Care is always taken when treating any woman who is between 12 and 14 weeks pregnant, as it is at this time that the placenta takes over from the ovaries in hormone production and the risk of miscarriage is greatest. Much of the low back pain and cramping experienced during pregnancy can be alleviated. As the pelvic changes take place later in the pregnancy, the foetus may become fixed on one side and create pain; this can be helped by the special techniques of Chiropractic. After pregnancy, as the body attempts to return to normality, often there is resulting back pain and a good spinal manipulation can be very helpful. The patient returns to her normal self much quicker and feels great benefit.

What to Expect from a Visit to a Chiropractor

At the initial consultation, the Chiropractor will take a detailed case history. This will give the Chiropractor information to help in the treatment he or she is about to give. The Chiropractor will then perform a physical orthopaedic examination, with various tests to make sure recovery under Chiropractic treatment will be certain. He or she will also feel or palpate the spine for any irregularities, tenderness, swellings, etc., to determine the most appropriate treatment. If the Chiropractor feels at this time that the patient needs an X-ray of the spine, this will be suggested. Many Chiropractors have their own equipment and are trained in its use and diagnosis. A spine is like a blueprint and is very individualistic. Each person is unique, therefore each patient's spine will be different even though the symptoms patients present may seem similar. If there is further doubt in the Chiropractor's mind further tests (blood, urine, etc.) may be suggested. After all findings are complete, the Chiropractor will then give the patient an explanation of the diagnosis and, should he or she feel unable to help, would refer the patient to a GP.

WHAT IS CHIROPRACTIC TREATMENT?

There are many techniques, from hard thrusts with the body to simple fast thrusts with the palm of the hand on the spine. Some may be heavy, others very light. New soft tissue techniques may be used on muscles and joints to relax and help relieve the spinal pressure. Applied Kinesiology or muscular techniques are frequently appropriate. Heavy or light massage to relax the spine and muscles may be employed. All this really depends on the age, diagnosis, chronicity or length of time of the condition, the amount of tenderness and what the Chiropractor feels the patient can tolerate. The treatment or adjustment maybe given on the patient's stomach, back or by a twisting motion to the patient's side.

The Chiropractor, with the knowledge gained from an examination and X-ray, is very specific in adjusting the segment needing realignment, therefore minimizing any reaction from the adjustment – in some chronic conditions the patient may not feel any change for several days or treatments. After the first treatment there could be a slight improvement, after the second treatment more relief and each further treatment should bring continued improvement. In general, the patient should not expect a cure at the first visit. Even though the pain may have started suddenly this does not necessarily mean that the condition started at the same time. Science has shown that, for instance, vertebral discs can build up stress and then, with the simplest wrong move, prolapse and pressure on the nerves can result, causing severe pain in the back. Sometimes this severe sudden pain brings the individual to his knees or to the floor. Many times I have visited patients at home and applied emergency treatment to enable them to visit the clinic. If after a reasonable period of treatment, which varies with each individual and the condition's complexities, there is no improvement, the patient will be referred to other practitioners.

However, in some cases, the old cliché that you have to get worse to get better may apply; in other cases a seemingly miraculous recovery can occur and a patient may get off the treatment couch feeling much better. As a general rule it will require, for back pain, an average of six treatments; in some cases it will take less but again in many of chronic severity it will take more. I have found in my practice that for maintenance purposes, a treatment every month or every three months is a good way to stay healthy. Prevention is far better than having to react to a painful and debilitating injury.

The time required to give treatment may be quite short, say 15 to 20 minutes. My old Professor said 'Find it, fix it and leave it alone, adjust the vertebrae, put your hands in your pockets and whistle. Let the innate natural healing power of the body do its job.' This says a lot, as no treatment actually heals; only the body and its inherent qualities is capable of healing. Everything outside the body only assists this magnificent process.

WHAT IS THE DIFFERENCE BETWEEN CHIROPRACTIC AND OSTEOPATHY?

In theory and application there are differences. Chiropractors use more diagnostic X-rays, therefore they are more specific in their choice of segment to adjust. Osteopaths use more leverage in adjustments, but both are similar manipulative techniques and achieve good results. Chiropractic interacts well with other therapies, especially those of a hands-on nature.

WHAT WILL MY GP SAY?

Many GPs are recognizing the value of spinal manipulation and refer patients to Chiropractors. The General Medical Council has given its permission to this end. This, of course, is in the best interest of the patient.

QUALIFICATIONS

There are about 17 Chiropractic colleges in the US and one in the UK (the Anglo-European College); Canada, Australia and France have one college each. These colleges offer full-time courses of four years' duration; on graduation they confer a degree of DC (Doctor of Chiropractic). These colleges also have a university status and may award a BSc degree which is also transferable to other universities of higher academic education. In the UK there is also an Institute of Pure Chiropractic which uses Open University lines in tandem with clinical training under one-to-one supervision. The British Chiropractic Association and the Institute of Pure Chiropractic are able to supply lists of registered members; registration is an assurance of a practitioner's ethical standard, qualifications and conduct.

The British Chiropractic Association
29 Whitley Street
Reading
Berkshire RG2 0EG

The Institute of Pure Chiropractic
150 Wroslyn Road
Freeland
Oxford
Oxfordshire OX8 8HL

USA
American Chiropractic Association
1701 Clarendon Blvd.
Arlington, VA 24203
Tel. 703–276–8800

Further Reading
Anthea Courtenay, *Chiropractic for Everyone* (Penguin Books, 1987)
Michael B. Howitt Wilson, *Thorsons Introductory Guide to Chiropractic* (Thorsons, 1991)

❧ Colour Healing ❧

ANGELA KIRK

Origins

Colour has played an important part in shaping our history. Primitive man associated colour with the life-force and considered it a mysterious power. As civilization developed, colour was used extensively, with an ever-wider range of materials becoming available. The ancient Egyptians were well aware of the powerful energies of colour as a healing agent in their temples. Through the ages humanity's thinking and attitudes have been reflected by its use of colour.

Nowadays the human eye can perceive about one thousand distinguishable hues and more than two thousand tints and shades. We naturally link colour with situations and places: red alerts us to danger, white is connected with doctors and healing centres, purple is synonymous with High Church and Royalty, while blue is often recognized as the colour of law and authority.

We automatically 'tune' in to colour and have an instinctive reaction to the shades we need to make us feel well and happy. Today, colour is used in a variety of ways: to tempt the shopper, influence our mood in the home or office, promote safety at work, help prevent crimes such as vandalism, and also to calm disturbed people in prisons and hospitals. The old sayings 'feeling blue', 'green with envy', 'seeing red' and 'in the pink' have more than a basis in truth. Colour not only influences the image we present, but also reflects and affects our health and emotions. These colour rays may be applied to the body either physically, through exposure to light rays themselves, or mentally, through techniques of suggestion, visualization or meditation. When we become diseased there is altered function which is the natural response of the body to strain. To restore our physical, mental or spiritual well-being, colour (made up of varying light/energy frequencies) may be applied.

HOW IT WORKS

All life begins and is sustained by light. We now know that visible light contains all colour and is a small part of the electromagnetic spectrum. Each of the bands of colour will have a different healing quality. Red has a long wavelength, slow vibration and is stimulating in action, while violet, at the other end of the spectrum, has a short wavelength, fast vibration and is subduing in action. Infra-red and ultra-violet are invisible rays at either end of the colour spectrum, yet can also be used as healing agents. The importance of full-spectrum (white or sun-) light has only recently been realized as people have been found to suffer from 'Seasonal Affective Disorder', more commonly known as winter depression. The body needs 15 minutes of sunlight a day to maintain health, otherwise the body can suffer from symptoms similar to those of jet-lag.

Around the body there is an electromagnetic field known as the *aura*. Throughout the ages, mystics and seers have seen the aura with psychic ability; painters have depicted this energy as a halo. In 1908, Semyon Kirlian managed to photograph this human energy.

All of us sense others' 'vibes' and know intuitively how other people are feeling. We have sayings such as 'birds of a feather flock together' and 'like attracts like', which can be interpreted to mean that the colours in the auras are compatible, while personality clashes indicate that the people who have very different colours in their aura will find it hard to understand each other.

The colours in someone's aura may be enhanced as he or she gradually makes progress and learns from the experiences of life. These colours will show the gifts and potential of a person as well as any area of negativity, which may be 'seen' psychically as dull or muddy colours due to wrong thinking. Strong colours may flash temporarily through the aura if the person is in a rage, or conversely full of love, so colours will indicate true feelings.

The body may be likened to a musical instrument. The spinal column represents the keyboard, with base notes being placed at the bottom of the spine. The colour spectrum ranges from red through to the 'top notes' of violet at the crown centre of the head.

WHAT TO EXPECT FROM A VISIT TO A THERAPIST

During our lives, the energy centres (or *chakras*) of the body need to be tuned by balancing the colours with right thinking and releasing negative energy, thereby restoring harmony and health. Within each chakra the life-force is both received and radiated, producing the auric colours that surround the body. Energy that is absorbed will affect the endocrine system and the nervous system.

When a client comes for a consultation, his or her energy field will be examined with clairvoyant sight to make a diagnosis. The colour therapist will suggest different ways to treat any colour deficiency. This might involve stepping up the intake of the right-colour foods or changing the decor of a room. As energy follows thought, meditation with creative visualization is often the best and most effective way of balancing our colours. The client will be taught deep relaxation techniques and may be taken on an imaginary journey which is full of colour. With the aid of suitable music, stress can be reduced and the person will feel revitalized.

CONDITIONS FOR WHICH IT IS EFFECTIVE

All the colours have positive and negative aspects; too much or too little will cause an imbalance in the system. In perfect health there should be an impartial liking for all the colours, since only by the equal blending can there be perfect harmony.

RED
Represents passion and energy, and is a strong stimulant. Very little red is used in colour healing because it can cause inflammation and the person may become over-excited or irritable. Small amounts, however, are particularly helpful in cases of anaemia and depression.

ORANGE
Has a freeing action on the body. It is one of the most frequently used colours in healing because it gives energy to the physical body and wisdom to the mind. It is useful in promoting self-confidence and heals nervous complaints.

YELLOW
Has a cleansing and purifying action on the body. It will stimulate a sluggish digestion and is the colour of joy and happiness. It will aid anyone studying for exams by enhancing concentration.

GREEN
Combines the yellow of wisdom with the blue of truth. Many invalids are sent to the country to recover from illness due to an instinctive knowledge that the green will act as a tonic and harmonizer. It is very beneficial for nervous complaints, and brings peace of mind and a clear memory.

BLUE
Is soothing and promotes healing. Many healers have this colour in

their aura. It will reduce fevers and blood pressure and will act as an antiseptic and pain-killer. It will help encourage acceptance of things that cannot be changed and bring peace of mind.

INDIGO

Calms the mind and is a great purifier. It helps in cases of migraine or any other painful conditions. This colour is used to enhance psychic development.

VIOLET

Is helpful for all nervous and mental disturbances and will be beneficial for lung disorders. If seen in the aura it will indicate a person with spiritual awareness.

A craving for – or even an aversion to – a particular colour is a sign that the body needs that particular wavelength. The rays we draw to ourselves, whether good or bad, will be re-radiated to others with whom we come into contact, so by harmonizing our colours we will enhance the light in the world.

Further Reading
Mary Anderson, *Colour Therapy* (Aquarian, 1990)

CRANIAL OSTEOPATHY

SIBYL GRUNDBERG

ORIGINS

Cranial Osteopathy may appear to be a New Age phenomenon, but in fact interest in this approach has been growing steadily for the last 60 years. In 1899 a bright Osteopathic student called William Garner Sutherland observed the potential for movement between the bones of the adult skull, which are separate at birth but come together during childhood. Ten years later, still haunted by his observation and still sceptical, he set out to prove that such movement was impossible, at first using bone specimens. Later came a series of experiments employing ingenious mechanical devices designed to compress his own head in specific ways. His severe reactions, both mental and physical, demonstrated not only motion involving the cranial bones, but also a deep, regular pulse throughout the body.

PHILOSOPHY

It is this slow fluid rhythm or respiration, which Sutherland called the Involuntary Mechanism, that forms the basis of Osteopathic work in the cranial field, an Osteopathic approach which takes into account the influence of cranial mechanics and fluid dynamics upon all the tissues of the body.

Andrew Taylor Still, Osteopathy's founder and primary theorist, stressed the importance of keeping the channels of blood, lymph and cerebrospinal fluid open, allowing all the body tissues to 'breathe' or absorb nutrients, as well as to eliminate waste products. Restrictions in the mobility of joints are known to lead to swelling and pressure, which block the health-giving interchange of fluid between these channels and adjacent cells. Dr Sutherland's contribution was to see the possibility of intervention in this process at a different level: releasing tensions by harnessing the body's own self-balancing and self-healing powers.

Where any part of the body is tight, painful and distressed, this will be reflected by a disturbed quality of the involuntary rhythm in that area – sometimes, as in severe head or spinal injuries, throughout the whole mechanism. Osteopaths use very gentle pressure and holding or easing techniques to alter disturbed patterns of movement. A rebalancing of tissue tensions follows.

WHAT TO EXPECT FROM A VISIT TO A THERAPIST

The Cranial Osteopath will use all available means to diagnose your condition with precision, including an interview, discussion of your medical history, and a physical examination which takes the whole body into account. This ensures both safety and the best chances of success in treatment. To assess the Involuntary Mechanism, the practitioner typically places both hands on the body, 'listening' for the pattern and quality of movement in various areas, including the cranium. You may feel very little while your Osteopath is working in this way; or you may feel, once treatment is underway, peace, warmth, or a very specific release of tension in the affected part.

Most people find treatment relaxing; a few may even be aware of rebalancing sensations occurring in their bodies. Treatment reactions (the temporary worsening of symptoms) occasionally occur, usually settling down within 24 or 48 hours. If you are worried about any of your responses to treatment, telephone your Osteopath.

Cranial Osteopaths may use other Osteopathic skills at appropriate points in a course of treatment; but each case is treated individually. Your Osteopath will be glad to answer your questions, and to discuss the method, aims and expectations of your treatment plan.

WHO CAN BENEFIT?

Osteopathy in the cranial field, sometimes called 'fluid Osteopathy', is a useful choice of treatment for people who require a gentle approach and for people with long-term pain and discomfort related to old physical injuries, including birth trauma. Children of all ages, particularly those under five years of age, respond very well to cranial treatment; indeed, some early childhood disorders which may not appear at first to be related to cranial compression at birth can be improved if treatment is given in these early years.

In cases of chronic pain, work with the cranial rhythmic impulse can prolong the effectiveness of Osteopathic treatment. For example, if a current problem is found to be related to an old injury, such treatment can produce complete, long-standing relief. It can also be helpful after recent violence, such as a road traffic accident, head injury or fracture – after appropriate conventional medical treatment – by releasing the effects of shock which may be 'locked' in the tissues.

HOW IT INTERACTS WITH OTHER THERAPIES

Cranial Osteopathy is usually compatible with a wide range of other treatments such as **Homoeopathy**, **Naturopathy** and

Herbal Medicine. If you are already having Acupuncture, Shiatsu, Polarity Therapy or Biodynamic Massage, it is a good idea to discuss the plan, and particularly the timing of treatments, with the practitioners involved.

People who like a gentle, relaxing treatment and who have, or who would like to have, a sense of their own deep self-balancing potential, will profit from the Cranial approach. 'Instant cures' can occur, but patience and commitment may be necessary in the progressive unlocking of long-standing body tensions. There is still work to be done in developing this powerful approach, but already Cranial Osteopathy has so much to offer the patient in the gentle release of pain and suffering.

QUALIFICATIONS

Strictly, there is no such thing as a 'Cranial Osteopath'. We are all simply Osteopaths who have a particular interest in the Involuntary Mechanism, and have undertaken years of training, study and practice in this approach. Although there is no separate register of Osteopaths trained to work in this way, they should be listed with the Register of Osteopaths as having done a four-year full-time (or a six-year part-time) course of clinical and Osteopathic studies, in which case they will have the letters DO, MRO after their name. However, after the British Government's Osteopaths' Bill of 1993 comes into effect – probably some time in 1995 – only those who have successfully undertaken the training recognized by the General Osteopathic Council will be able to call themselves Osteopaths.

General Council and Register of Osteopaths
56 London Road
Reading
Berkshire RG1 4SQ
Tel. 0734 576585

The GCRO will refer patients to members of The Sutherland Society, a national network of Osteopaths who have trained in working with the cranial approach.

The Osteopathic Centre for Children
4 Harcourt House
19a Cavendish Square
London W1M 9AD
Tel. 071–495 1231

Australia & New Zealand
Sutherland Cranial Teaching Foundation of Australia & New
    Zealand
Hillside Health Centre
2 Hillside Parade
Glen Iris
Melbourne
Victoria 3146
Tel. (61) 3 889 6767

USA
The Cranial Academy
3500 DePauw Boulevard #1080
Indianapolis, IN 46268–1139
Tel. 317–879–0713
Fax 317–879–0718

Further Reading

Ada Strand Sutherland, *With Thinking Fingers* (Indianapolis: The Cranial Academy, 1962). *Sutherland's life and work, written by his widow.*

William Garner Sutherland, *The Cranial Bowl* (pamphlet available from The Cranial Academy, 1939)

These books are available in the UK from Osteopathic Supplies, 70 Belmont Road, Hereford HR2 7JW.

✎ Homoeopathy ✎

PETER FINEGAN

Origins

To introduce Homoeopathy properly we must go back some 200 years and look at one of the most fascinating stories in medical history. It is a story of one man's discovery of the principles of Homoeopathy, and his inspired thinking at a time when medicine was static in its approaches to illness.

The man who stands centre-stage in this story is Samuel Hahnemann, a German doctor who in 1786 was a prominent physician and medical author. As a young physician his reputation in both chemistry and medicine grew widely, and he was soon established at the top of his profession. However, the practice of medicine in its form at that time did not sit well with him. As he wrote to a friend in 1796,

> *It was agony for me to walk always in darkness, when I had to heal the sick according to such and such an hypothesis concerning diseases or substances which owed their place in the* Materia Medica *to an arbitrary decision...*

On another occasion he also wrote,

> *I renounced the practice of medicine, that I might no longer incur the risk of doing injury, and I engaged in chemistry exclusively and in literary occupations.*

It was at this stage of Hahnemann's life, faced with disillusionment in his medical work, that he turned his attention exclusively to translating medical texts and to studying the *Materia Medica*. This was the turning point in his life and the start of a new way of thinking which would eventually be known as Homoeopathy.

Hahnemann relentlessly probed into both historical and contemporary ideas about health and disease; his enthusiasm and will brought him finally to the edge of his great discovery. Around the year 1800, while translating the *Materia Medica* (a text concerning the actions and therapeutic effects of substances) written by Professor Cullen of London University, he came across a part of the text devoted to the therapeutic indications of Peruvian Bark (a source of what is known today as quinine). In his *Materia Medica*, Cullen attributed its success in the treatment of malaria to the fact that it was bitter-tasting. Hahnemann found this explanation both vague and irritating to his scientific mind, so much so that he did something unusual. He took a series of doses of Peruvian Bark himself. It was the action of a man whose approach to medicine was in keeping with this extraordinary experiment. He described the results as follows:

> *I took by way of experiment, twice a day four drachms of good China (Peruvian Bark). My feet, finger ends etc. at first became cold; I grew languid and drowsy; then my heart began to palpitate, and my pulse grew hard and slow; then pulsation in the head, redness of the cheeks, thirst, and, in short all these symptoms, which are ordinarily characteristic of intermittent fever (malaria) made their appearance, one after the other, yet without the peculiar chilly shivering rigor. This paroxysm lasted two or three hours each time, and recurred if I repeated this dose, not otherwise. I discontinued it, and was in good health.*

This was indeed a revelation to Hahnemann, as he had actively discovered that a drug which was known to be curative in malaria actually produced the very symptoms of the condition when taken by a healthy person. He accepted this observation as the basis of the reason why all substances have a therapeutic action on an illness, and went on to make further experiments and 'prove' the action of other substances. He summed up his new discovery by saying,

A substance which produces symptoms in a healthy person cures those same symptoms in a sick person.

This formed the basis of his 'Law of Similars' which to this day underpins all Homoeopathic thinking.

Hahnemann's discoveries began to attract other doctors to his new way of thinking, colleagues who, like himself, were looking further than the ideas of the medical establishment of the day. Over the next five years they systematically experimented upon themselves in the same way Hahnemann had originally done, using many different substances. Over this period Hahnemann also compiled a list of accidental poisonings recorded by different doctors throughout Europe. The symptoms produced by poisons and those by the experiments done by this small group were gathered together, and of course he and his colleagues recognized in them the identical symptom pictures of many illnesses which they were accustomed to seeing in their practices, many of which were considered incurable.

Hahnemann called his new medicine Homoeopathy, a word taken from the Greek 'Omeos' meaning similar and 'Pathos' meaning suffering. Thus Homoeopathy's meaning is to 'treat with something that produces an effect similar to the suffering'.

It was a logical next step for Hahnemann and his colleagues to begin treating sick people using this new approach. They found that the results were as exciting as their original discoveries had suggested they would be. They began to have great success in treating illnesses which up till that time had been understood to be difficult to manage. It was at this point that Hahnemann moved on to his next discovery.

While he was treating his patients with Homoeopathy he began to see that initially patients were over-stimulated by the substances he was using, producing aggravations. He quickly realized that the actual amount given a patient was all-important and began to experiment with reducing the dosage. He reduced the dose to one tenth of its usual amount and found that the patient was cured but the aggravation, though slighter, remained. He diluted further, each time prescribing one tenth of the previous dose, and finally reached a dilution that was ineffective. He came to the belief that if the medicine were not strong enough to aggravate the symptoms, it would be ineffective in bringing about a cure.

At this critical stage, Hahnemann once again made a crucial discovery. He found that by strongly shaking the medicine at each dilution, or 'succussing' it (as he called this process), it became not only less toxic but actually more potent and therefore more likely to bring about a cure in the patient. The implications of this discovery were amazing. Once more he had crossed a threshold of knowledge and reached a new understanding. Homoeopaths to this present day demonstrate this discovery time and time again in giving substances which are diluted to levels of one part per million and beyond and still bringing about a cure in the patient.

What Hahnemann concluded was that in every substance in nature there lay hidden an inner 'vital force' or 'life', which could be used to potentiate healing. It was this, he concluded, which 'acted' therapeutically, stimulating the person's own 'vital force' or 'life energy' to bring about well-being.

It should not be surprising that Hahnemann met with disbelief and prejudiced opinion among his peer group. Even in the 20th century, with the advent of modern Physics and its understanding of atomic structures and energy potentials within matter, there are many within the establishment of medicine who still view Hahnemann's discoveries with prejudice and scepticism.

PHILOSOPHY

As Hahnemann's work progressed and his understanding deepened he began to draw together his ideas in his writings, especially in his book *The Organon of the Art of Healing* written in about 1810. In this book he wrote extensively on his findings and outlined the basis of Homoeopathic thinking. He maintained that:

1. A substance which produces symptoms in a healthy person cures those symptoms in a sick person.
2. The dynamic vital force is primarily affected in an individual who is sick, and therefore the medicine itself must be able to affect this by being itself dynamic.
3. The patient only needs one particular medicine at a time.
4. The totality of symptoms is what must be prescribed on, or a remedy found for.

This last law we will look at in a little more depth, as it will help the reader to understand how a Homoeopath works. In asserting that the *total symptom picture* was paramount in the matching of the symptoms to the medicine, Hahnemann was embracing what today is known as a holistic view of the illness. If we backtrack for a moment, and look at Hahnemann and his colleagues' early work, what we find is that their 'provings' of these substances, i.e. the symptoms gathered from the taking of these agents and the study of poisonings, showed symptoms at the physical, emotional and mental level. For instance, in the proving of *Lycopodium clavatum* (club moss) it was noted that physical symptoms occurred often on the right side of the body, and that the digestive system was greatly affected with distension, gas and pain. Also, however, the affected person would be anxious, develop a fear of being alone and would be worse between the hours of 4 and 8 p.m. To Hahnemann, then, symptoms which before had often been overlooked became crucial in deciding which remedy would be 'similar' and therefore curative to a patient's illness – in this case, Club Moss was found to be helpful in treating Irritable Bowel Syndrome among other conditions.

What to Expect from a Visit to a Homoeopath

In keeping with the 'totality of symptoms' law, a Homoeopath will be interested in all of the patient's symptoms however minor or unimportant he or she may feel them to be. A case history will be detailed, with the aim of finding out if the patient is better or worse under certain circumstances or times of the day, in different temperatures and conditions and so on. The Homoeopath will ask about the temperament of the patient, whether he or she is timid, irritable, anxious, fearful, etc. He will want to know about diet and food desires or aversions, as well as sleep patterns, temperature reactions, etc. Slowly a thorough picture is built up by the Homoeopath of the symptom pattern and general constitutional state of the patient. As a final stage, this symptom pattern will be compared to the most similar medicine in the *Materia Medica* of provings; it is this medicine (given in the appropriate strength) which will be the curative agent.

A cure was said by Hahnemann to be at best 'slow, gentle and permanent'. While aggravations of symptoms may occur in Homoeopathy, these should be minimal and in many cases absent if the correct dosage is used. Cure most often occurs from inside the patient, and many times the physical symptoms are the last to disappear. In these cases the patient may first report feeling like his or her 'old self' again; and finally, over time, report that the physical complaint has cleared up as well.

Samuel Hahnemann not only discovered a new approach to the healing of the sick, which he called Homoeopathy, but he also gave humanity a method of curing illness which since the end of his life has grown 'slowly, gently and permanently' to every continent on Earth, and in its time has given back millions of people the health and well-being which they sought. It is my belief it will find its true place at the forefront of medicine in the 21st century.

HOW IT FITS INTO AN INDIVIDUAL'S LIFESTYLE

Homoeopathic remedies are prescribed in pill form which dissolve readily in the mouth. Nothing should be taken by mouth for 20 minutes before or after a remedy (including toothpaste or drinks). You may be asked to refrain from drinking coffee or eating peppermints during a course of treatment, as either can adversely effect the remedy. Remedies should also be stored away from strong-smelling substances e.g. perfumes, camphor or eucalyptus, as these can inhibit the effect of the remedy. Before embarking on any other form of treatment it is best to check with your Homoeopath first – even dental work can affect the action of remedies.

Generally, follow-up treatment after an initial consultation is likely to be at monthly intervals, to assess the progress made, but depending on the severity of symptoms this may be more frequent if appropriate. The length of time taken to effect a cure is difficult to predict, as each person responds to treatment in an individualistic way. However, acute, short-term problems do not require lengthy treatment, while conditions of long standing will take longer to clear.

CONDITIONS FOR WHICH IT IS EFFECTIVE

Due to its wide-ranging effect on physical, mental and emotional states, Homoeopathic treatment can address a broad spectrum of conditions, too numerous to list here. Structural problems are best dealt with by a structural therapist (for example a Chiropractor or Osteopath), but apart from that Homoeopathy has an extremely broad approach. If in doubt, a short talk to a practitioner will clarify whether your condition is suited to Homoeopathic treatment.

Common everyday accidents and problems such as burns, bruises, stings, sprains, stomach upsets, pre-exam nerves, emotional shock, trauma, etc. can be easily treated with first-aid Homoeopathic remedies which can safely be kept at home and administered either under the guidance of a Homoeopath or after some short study of the subject; this often rules out the need for the use of more expensive synthetic drugs.

WHO CAN BENEFIT?

Because of its broad base Homoeopathy is suitable for all ages, from babies through to the elderly. Because of its gentle action, freedom from side-effects and its easy administration anyone can benefit. Babies and young children respond particularly well; treatment is non-invasive and is not traumatic and will address common childhood illnesses, ear, nose and throat problems, skin conditions, behavioural problems, etc. Elderly people with rheumatic complaints, arthritis, insomnia, circulatory or digestive problems and many more also respond well to this gentle form of treatment. Pregnant women benefit and certain remedies are particularly effective during both pregnancy and labour, often ruling out the need for stronger conventional drugs which can affect the baby. Even animals respond positively. The treatment and positive response of animals has discounted the theory put about by sceptics that Homoeopathic remedies owe nothing more to their success than the placebo effect.

HOW IT INTERACTS WITH OTHER THERAPIES

Some therapies are compatible with Homoeopathic treatment, but others should be avoided. If, for instance, you are being treated by a Homoeopath but also have a structural problem, you may be referred to see an Osteopath or Chiropractor (**Chiropractic**), or an **Alexander Technique** practitioner. Other main therapies, for example Acupuncture, Herbal treatment and Polarity Therapy, should not be combined with Homoeopathic treatment, as it becomes increasingly difficult to ascertain which treatment is creating what effect and the whole issue becomes clouded. Aromatherapy, because of its use of essential oils, is also incompatible because the strong-smelling oils nullify the effects of the remedies. The best policy is always to seek the advice of the Homoeopath before embarking on any other form of treatment.

QUALIFICATIONS

Some GPs are trained Homoeopaths and use it within their medical practice. As Homoeopathic medicine is recognized in the UK by Act of Parliament, treatment is available on the National Health Service, at hospitals in London, Glasgow, Liverpool, Bristol and Kent. A list of medical practitioners is available from The British Homoeopathic Association (see address below).

The Society of Homoeopaths (address below) is the professional body for non-medically qualified Homoeopaths. Members of their register have to follow a strict code of ethics and are examined by the Society as to their competence. There are many Homoeopathic training establishments throughout Britain. Courses are generally lengthy and their curriculum has to fulfil certain criteria governed by the Society of Homoeopaths in order to be recognized training establishments.

In order to find a Homoeopath in your area the following addresses will be useful:

The British Homoeopathic Association
27a Devonshire Street
London WC1N 1RJ
Tel. 071–935 2163

The Hahnemann Society
Humane Education Centre
Bounds Green Road
London N22 4EV
Tel. 081–889 1595

The Society of Homoeopaths
2 Artizan Road
Northampton NN1 4HV
Tel. 0604 21400

Australia
Australian Federation of Homoeopaths
21 Bulah Close
Berowra Heights
NSW 2082
Tel. 02 456 3602

USA
National Center for Homoeopathy
801 N. Fairfax Street
Alexandria, VA 22314
Tel. 703–548–7790

Further Reading

Anne Clover, *Thorsons Introductory Guide to Homoeopathy* (Thorsons, 1991)

Harold Gaier, *Thorsons Encyclopaedic Dictionary of Homoeopathy* (Thorsons, 1991)

Samuel Hahnemann, *Organon of Medicine* (Los Angeles: J. P. Tarcher, 1982 [first published 1810])

Herbert A. Roberts, *Principles and Art of Cure by Homoeopathy* (Homoeopathic Publishing Co, 1936)

George Vithoulkas, *Medicine of the New Man* (New York: Arco, 1979)

—, *The Science of Homoeopathy* (Thorsons, 1986)

๑ HYPNOTHERAPY ๑

KIRSTI E. HOLM

ORIGINS

The history of hypnosis goes back to ancient times; it was used as a cure by early civilizations such as those of the ancient Egyptians, Persians, Greeks and Romans. In Athens, at the base of the southern slope of Acropolis, lie the ruins of the temple of Asklepios. There, those for whom physical illness or soul sickness had persevered, despite all human efforts at healing, would prepare to be treated by the gods. After a ritual cleansing, the sick person would be led to the innermost sanctuary to lie on a couch, where the god of sleep, *Hypnos*, and the god of dreams *Oneiros*, had their statues. The treatment consisted of sleeping and dreaming until a dream occurred which healed the patient.

Over the centuries, this basic architecture of clinical treatment for troubles of the body and soul, the soma and psyche has remained, even while the stones of the temple crumbled. We can see the same arches and columns in the modern practice of psychology and hypnosis, for psychology is 'knowledge of the soul' and hypnosis 'a condition like sleep'.

From time to time over the last two centuries, various people have developed methods that have depended on hypnosis. The Austrian doctor Franz Anton Mesmer found that he was able to cure people of different diseases without medicines or surgery; despite much controversy regarding these techniques his name remains with us as a common term: to be mesmerized, meaning, that we are completely fascinated or as if under a 'spell'.

Throughout the second half of the 19th century hypnosis was

studied and taught by an increasing number of doctors in Britain and France. One of the best known was Sigmund Freud, who studied hypnosis under the French neurologist Jean-Martin Charcot. Initially Freud used hypnosis to enhance the effects of suggestions he would make to remove patients' psychiatric symptoms. Later he became more and more convinced that psychiatric symptoms often represented memories, feelings and inner conflicts of which the patient was not conscious, so he began to use hypnosis to investigate the subconscious mind. Although these methods often seemed to produce satisfactory improvements in the condition of the patients, the effects were often short-lived. What Freud did not fully appreciate was that an essential factor for success was the co-operation of the patient. When, in some cases, this co-operation was lacking and the expected cure did not take place, Freud concluded that hypnosis was not an appropriate mode of treatment and conceived the technique of 'free association' as a means of gaining access to the subconscious memories, feelings and thoughts of his patients. With hindsight we find that the technique he developed is more closely related to hypnosis as it is practised today, although it was very different from the hypnotic methods of his own time.

In the last 30 years there has been a vast improvement in the hypnotic techniques used as a method of healing mental and physical problems. The principles of modern Hypnotherapy are based on the unusual and innovative methods of the late Dr Milton H. Erickson, an American psychiatrist who pioneered modern hypnosis, a methodology that is completely different from the more traditional 'authoritarian' hypnosis. Erickson was a creative genius who devised many unusual and beneficial therapy methods. The most up-to-date hypnotic techniques have followed on from his work.

PHILOSOPHY

Hypnosis is a perfectly natural phenomenon. It is just like sleep, yet a hypnotic trance is not sleep (though sometimes hypnosis seems to resemble it). The hypnotic trance is essentially a state of deep absorption. In simple terms, it is nothing more (and nothing less) than a special state of altered awareness, achieved usually with the aid of another person, although, of course, it can be self-induced.

The hypnotic trance state is very familiar to us; we all undergo trances from time to time – when we are pre-occupied with what we are doing, for example. When we are completely absorbed in music, memory, day-dreaming or watching a play or a film, we can lose touch with our surroundings and not notice the passage of time. These are everyday examples of natural trance states. It is the utilization of this trance state, this altered state of awareness, which is used to build in the mind ideas of self-improvement and desired changes of behaviour, etc. Because one is away from the distractions of everyday life, one's state of altered awareness will have a special quality, which varies from person to person.

The brain is the body's most miraculous possession, the seat of intellect and sensation. It works silently, directing every single thing we do: the thoughts we have, the movements we make and the delicate bodily functions which keep us alive. It determines who we are. But how well do we use it? Every single experience, thought and idea we have ever had, every hope and projection for the future, every feeling about the present, are all stored in our brains at this moment as memories, and when conditions are right all these memories can be retrieved!

The brain has two hemispheres, the right and the left; in the centre is the *corpus callosum*. The left hemisphere, the conscious mind, is the reasoning mind; the right hemisphere is the subconscious mind which accepts what is impressed upon it without any judgement (for people who are left-handed, the opposite is the case). Different activities take place in different parts of the brain:

Left Hemisphere	Right Hemisphere
Consciousness	Unconsciousness
Logic	Recognition
Reason	Rhythm
Mathematics	Visualization
Language	Creativity
Reading	Synthesis
Writing	Dreaming
Analysis	Symbolic thought
Ego	Emotions
	Id

In hypnosis, activities in the two hemispheres can take place freely; the gate is opened between the two. We spend our lives doing what we feel like doing or what we intellectually have to do. When the feeling mind and the intellectual mind are in conflict, the feeling mind usually wins. Sometimes the intellect may overrule the feelings to avoid painful consequences. For example, in the case of overeating or smoking, the intellect knows this behaviour is destructive but the feelings win, and we continue to eat or smoke because it makes us feel good or temporarily stops us from feeling bad. When the intellect takes over violently to compress feelings, the imaginative function can become intensely negative, leading to feelings of hopelessness. The imagination is our source of hope. Einstein believed that he thought best in images, not words, and trusted his tremendously powerful instinctive imaginings. His theory of relativity began when he imagined what it would be like to ride a shaft of light into outer space. 'Imagination', he said 'is more important than knowledge.'

Hypnotherapy aims to bring our feeling and subconscious mind into alignment with our intellectual and conscious mind. We can imagine the coming together of elements in our lives that will bring us happiness by helping us to fill our deepest needs. In hypnotic trance, suggestions of self-improvement and desired changes in behaviour can be impressed on the subconscious mind.

The aim of Hypnotherapy is also to help a person focus and search inwardly, to utilize all his or her learning and skills to resolve problems, and to do so with the aid of subconscious learning and understanding.

WHAT TO EXPECT FROM A VISIT TO A HYPNOTHERAPIST

Hypnotherapy is based on respect for the client as a whole, in all the complexity and unique experience that makes us who we are. Hence Hypnotherapy does not impose a behaviour with which the client would not normally agree, but it does support and reinforce changes which have been consciously considered and which the client has decided are desirable.

Modern Hypnotherapy bears little relation to the popular presentation of stage hypnosis. For some people hypnosis is still shrouded in mystery and the swaying of pocket watches, an idea the professionals would like to reverse, as serious therapists have respect for and care about their clients. A good therapist is highly skilled in observation and is able to recognize even minor variations in behaviour that provide very important clues to a person's interests and abilities. These signs are utilized to help guide the client into the absorbing state of altered awareness that is generally called trance.

The skilled therapist has many ways of reaching the subconscious mind: these might include story-telling, inducing dreams, giving suggestions, leading the client through relaxation techniques, fantasy, life-scan, age regression, and so on. By turning the attention inward the person finds more of the self; this 'more of the self' is the subconscious mind. In hypnosis the client will not inadvertently reveal secrets – trance does not compel one to tell the truth and everything about oneself. Clients reveal only what they feel they can, at their own pace and in their own time. Normally the therapist does most of the talking while the client is in the trance state.

The client should be prepared to co-operate with the therapist and allow him- or herself to be hypnotized. Because each person is different, the depth of trance can vary from a light shallow state to a very deep state. Beneficial change can be effected even in the very shallow state. Contrary to popular belief, hypnosis does not have to be a state of complete relaxation. Deep trance is only one of the tools of advanced hypnotherapy; there are many avenues of approach to the subconscious mind that may be taken in order to overcome problems or achieve personal growth.

Some people are worried that they may be suspended in the trance state, but this cannot happen; the trance state is a very natural phenomenon and, if left undisturbed, the person in the trance would either fall into ordinary sleep and awaken soon after, or would just open his or her eyes and be fully aware again.

If you are considering Hypnotherapy, you may want to know how many sessions you would be expected to attend. This is always a difficult question to answer because we have to bear in mind that it is the whole person who presents for assistance; not just a set of 'symptoms' or 'aims'. We have been strongly conditioned to believe that change is slow and usually painful. Therapists using modern methods have found that this need not be so and that it is possible to make deep and lasting changes comparatively quickly and easily. We are all unique individuals and must be treated as such on all levels. However, the client should be aware of some positive progress, which does not always mean a complete cure, after four visits. If this is not happening then it might be wise either to change the therapist or the therapy.

WHO CAN BENEFIT?

The power of the subconscious mind is enormous; it has infinite intelligence and boundless wisdom. Whatever you impress upon your subconscious mind, it will move heaven and earth to bring to pass. We get used to relying on our rational faculties in everyday life, tending to neglect the bizarre and unconventional thoughts that arise from the emotional and imaginative side of our minds. However, these are just as valuable; they give us our most creative insights and the most inventive solutions to our problems, and enliven the daily grind.

Creativity is not simply an attribute some people are born with which enables them to produce works of art. Creativity gives us all more effective ideas to expand our options both at work and at home. It ensures we do not spend our lives running along tramlines but are innovative, flexible and ready to adapt to change. When we develop our creative ability, we start to find fresh solutions to the problems that face us. Take any problem: you can probably immediately come up with two or three options about how to deal with it. If you start to think creatively and use your subconscious mind, you may come up with 10 or 20.

Visual imagery has emerged as crucial to the creative process. The image in the mind's eye is not passive, as you might think, but active and can operate on other abstract ideas to create new concepts. The more vivid and spontaneous the pictures in the mind's eye are, the more the person's thinking diverges from the ordinary.

CONDITIONS FOR WHICH IT IS EFFECTIVE

As you now can imagine, there is no limit to the problems that can be treated effectively with Hypnotherapy. Each person has the solution to his or her own problem; the therapist is merely the catalyst. Having said this, we can mention a few specific problems for which hypnotherapy is particularly effective: lack of confidence, mental/emotional trauma, anxiety, depression, insomnia, phobias, obsessive or compulsive behaviour, unwanted habits (nail biting, thumb-sucking, stammering, blushing, smoking), eating disorders, infertility, impotence, pain control, high blood pressure, migraine, asthma and cancer. These are just a few of the many that could be listed. Additionally, clients often request the help of Hypnotherapy as an aid to personal growth, or to improve already adequate levels of performance in the areas of creativity, sport or decision-making. Help with relaxation, learning to visualize and self-hypnosis are also sought, sometimes by people who feel they have progressed a little way and then encounter difficulties while doing it on their own.

For Hypnotherapy to be effective a certain intelligence is required, so it would not be suitable for people with a learning or mental disability, or for young children.

How Hypnotherapy Interacts with Other Therapies

Hypnotherapy employs an understanding of people which is founded on the idea that anything that happens in the body also happens in the mind. Every thought or feeling we experience is manifested or shown in some bodily change or action. Similarly, every process in the body, or anything that happens to it, will necessarily have mental aspects, that is perceptions, thoughts and feelings associated with it.

When working in this way, therefore, Hypnotherapists believe that by using mental processes to produce changes in the mind, we are necessarily creating changes in the body also. The same, of course, is true the other way round: if we approach a person with physical treatments, mental changes will occur. A broken leg is not just a physical event in the body, but an event in the whole person.

Therefore, therapies such as **Acupuncture, Aromatherapy, Homoeopathy, Reflexology, (Cranial) Osteopathy** and **Nutritional Therapy**, etc. will work very well in conjunction with Hypnotherapy.

The modern methods of Hypnotherapy make use of a variety of therapeutic techniques both in and out of trance. Many of these techniques are borrowed from other schools of **Psychotherapy**. In the US there are 140 different therapies registered as Psychotherapy, and a great number of these are also used in Britain.

QUALIFICATIONS

There has never been a formal opinion in either the US or Britain that the occupational title 'Hypnotherapist' is restricted to those holding a licence in the healing arts or counselling professions.

This situation may change in Britain when it becomes fully integrated into the EC. In European countries some medical qualifications are required in order to practise hypnotherapy, but these requirements vary from country to country.

Central Register of Advanced Hypnotherapists
28 Finsbury Park Road
London N4 2JX

The National College of Hypnosis & Psychotherapy
12 Cross Street
Nelson
Lancashire

National Council of Psychotherapists & Hypnotherapy
Register
46 Oxhey Road
Oxhey
Watford WD1 4QQ

National Register of Hypnotherapists & Psychotherapists
12 Cross Street
Nelson
Lancashire

Further Reading

Valerie Austin, *Self-hypnosis* (Thorsons, 1994)

Helmut W. A. Karle, *Thorsons Introductory Guide to Hypnotherapy* (Thorsons, 1992)

❧ IRIDOLOGY ❧

SUE EVANS

Iridology – examination of the iris of the eye in order to analyse a person's state of health – is not a therapy as such but is a powerful tool which can be used by any therapist to gain deeper understanding of a patient's health and any underlying causes for disease. Iridology has been termed a diagnostic tool but it would perhaps be more accurate to term it analytic rather than diagnostic. The Iridologist can assess the condition of the tissues rather than name specific diseases. Inflammation, over-activity, congestion, toxic build-up and underfunction can all be determined from the iris. A spinal misalignment may show up in the iris, revealing the cause of disturbed tissue function to be either inadequate nerve supply or blockage of circulation and tissue drainage due to pressure from the displaced structures. A tendency for endocrine imbalance or a constitutional need for certain nutrients may be observed from the structural pattern of the iris fibres and variations in iris colour – and thus, not only can a complete picture be built up of the causes underlying a current health problem, but advice can be given on what an individual patient needs to maintain the best possible levels of health.

Imbalances in the body can show in the iris long before there are any clinical manifestations of disease. Iris analysis, or Ophthalmic Somatology as it is also termed, can be used preventatively in this way. By pinpointing the inherited strengths and weaknesses of the body, together with analysing the causes for acquired imbalances which are beginning to be revealed, a patient can be directed towards correct dietary, lifestyle and other measures to restore and maintain optimum health.

ORIGINS

The origins of iridology can be traced back as far as the Chaldean civilization, where carvings on a stone tablet make reference to its practice. It was certainly known among the early civilizations, although much of this knowledge has been lost to us, possibly due to the fact that, before the advent of high-resolution magnifying lenses and fine-beam torches, the application in the brown-eyed races was limited (the pigment in brown eyes covers many of the markings seen in the blue/grey iris). However, analysis is now equally possible for all people although it may require differing techniques and perhaps the accompaniment of analytical techniques such as pulse diagnosis.

Our present-day knowledge of iridology dates back to 1670, when Phillipus Meyens brought us one of our first published works on the subject. His work *Chiromatica Medica* describes the locations of the various parts of the body as they are reflected in the iris. It is, however, the Hungarian Dr Ignatz von Peczeley who is credited with being the 'Father' of Iridology. The story is told of how, as a young boy, he caught an owl in the garden, accidentally breaking its leg. As a result of this incident he noticed a marking appear in the bird's iris, which later faded as the leg healed to leave only a small dark imprint as evidence of the original fracture. The boy grew up to be a respected doctor, but this early incident had made such an impression on him that it led to a lifetime's study of the iris and its markings.

Von Peczeley's first chart of the iris, based on clinical observation, was published in 1881. The work seemed to gain momentum and more independent workers published the results of their research. Throughout Europe over the next 50 years iris charts were developed – by Liljequest in Sweden, Pastor Falke and his students in Germany, in the US by the Austrian-born Henry Lake (or Lane as he is sometimes known) and Dr Lindlahr, to name but a few. Although many charts have been produced, based largely on von Peczeley's model, one of the simplest and most widely known is that of a Dr Jensen, himself a student of Dr Lindlahr. Although it does not approach the complexity and intricate detail of the German charts, for example, it remains a good working model and allows a fine-tuned analysis to be made.

HOW IT WORKS

With the upsurge of interest in such disciplines as Reflexology and Ear Acupuncture, we are becoming accustomed to the concept that a small and seemingly unrelated area of the body can reflect and affect conditions elsewhere in the system. How is it then that Iridology works? In the developing embryo the eye grows out as an extension of the forebrain. Although developing as a specialized organ of sight, the eye remains, in essence, part of the brain; like the brain the iris receives impulses from all over the body, giving an up-to-the-minute account of prevailing conditions. Our skill at interpreting this information obviously falls far short of the wealth of information provided, but even within our own limitations, Iridologists still have an excellent, accurate and non-invasive analytical tool at our disposal.

While on the subject of limitations, however, let us state that there are certain things Iridology *cannot* do. Where an operation has been performed under anaesthetic the iris will retain no record of the surgery since nerve impulses will have been blocked. Where an organ has been removed the iris will retain the last recorded readings received from that organ. Irritation and congestion of the gall bladder together with other signs in the iris may lead one to deduce that gall stones are present, but an Iridologist will not be able to determine accurately the presence of gall or kidney stones. In our present state of knowledge we can, in some cases, note a predisposition to cancer and its most likely site of occurrence, but we cannot categorically determine whether a cancerous condition does or does not exist. Similarly we cannot tell if patients have HIV – as mentioned before, Iridology does not name diseases – all that could be said in such cases would be that there was a weakening and imbalance of the immune system. Iridology cannot determine pregnancy.

WHAT TO EXPECT FROM A VISIT TO A THERAPIST

For these reasons an Iridologist will usually take a detailed case history at some stage in the consultation. Symptoms experienced by the patient will be noted and, usually, other confirmatory analytical techniques may be used by the practitioner. Practice varies as to whether this is done before or after the iris examination, some practitioners preferring not to be unduly influenced by preconceptions arising from the case-taking, although others do not consider them a barrier to accurate iris analysis.

Examination of the iris may be achieved by use of a hand-held magnifying lens and torch or, in larger clinics, by a slit lamp or an iris camera. It is best to be aware that an iris photograph alone can be misleading due to various photographic effects and lack of certainty as to the exact axis of the iris. Practitioners will thus normally examine the iris with a lens and torch as well, keeping the photograph only for further clarification if necessary.

Most Iridologists will also be trained in at least one therapy so that they will be able to offer treatment if it falls within their sphere of practice. Sometimes a referral is necessary, for example to an Osteopath if the problem is structural, or even, if symptoms warrant, to a GP for further tests. A referral to a GP does not automatically mean that something is terribly wrong but may be used in order to eliminate certain possibilities before a practitioner can proceed with confidence. Blood tests may also be useful to confirm analysis and to monitor progress of treatment.

How it Interacts with Other Therapies

As previously mentioned, Iridology can be used with any discipline. Not only can it be used to analyse the cause of illness, but it can also monitor the return to health as signs of congestion and underfunction clear and lighten in the eye. Often these changes can be used to predict the onset of a 'healing crisis' – a short, acute phase that heralds the elimination of toxic residues and the return to higher levels of health. If ever a treatment is suppressive – such as the misuse or overuse of antibiotics, or the use of hydrocortisone creams for skin problems – this also will become apparent from the iris as the signs of congestion and underfunction will deepen rather than dispel, indicating a movement inward of the focus of disease. For this reason suppressive treatment is entirely at odds with the concepts and practice of Iridology.

Qualifications

There are two main schools of Iridology in Britain:

- The College of Ophthalmic Somatology – confers the initials MCOS or FCOS on its graduates.
- The Society of Iridology – RIr (Registered Iridologist)

Anyone bearing these initials is guaranteed to have received at least one year's in-depth tuition in iris analysis. Shortly, the initials IFI (belonging to the newly emergent International Federation of Iridologists) may also be awarded. The IFI accepts members both from within and outside the UK; its screening methods are rigorous and only well-qualified practitioners will be represented on its lists.

The College of Ophthalmic Somatology
28 Chapel Market
London N1 9EZ

International Federation of Iridologists
c/o Vicki Pitman
Hayes Corner
South Cheriton
Templecombe
Somerset BA8 0BR

The Society of Iridology
40 Storwood Road
Bournemouth BH3 7NE

Further Reading
Dorothy Hall, *Iridology* (Angus & Robertson, 1980)
Bernard Jensen, *Iridology Simplified* (Escondido, CA: B. Jensen, 1980)
Theodore Kriege, *Disease Signs in the Iris* (Romford: L. N. Fowler & Co., 1985)
Farida Sharan, *The Eyes of the World* (Saffron Walden: C. W. Daniel, 1989)

❧ NATUROPATHY ❧

JANET PROWER

ORIGINS

Naturopathy – or, as it is also known, Natural Therapeutics, Natural Medicine or Natural Hygiene – is an umbrella term covering that self-healing mechanism of the body which is automatically in harmony with nature. Man has always used nature to heal himself, more often by accident than by design. Naturopathy as it is practised today emulates the healing qualities of nature as used in the past: fasting was often used to give the body a chance to rest and throw off toxic wastes; different foods or plants were known to revitalize the various organs and systems of the body; sea water, hot springs and rivers have long been used to relieve aches and pains and help restore vitality and vigour; the peace and calm which comes from relaxation or meditation have been known and practised by many ancient societies. There is now a move to return to these simple truths.

The first Naturopaths, such as Lindlahr, Stanley Leif and Vogel, realized that man's health depended on being in harmony with nature and the Universe, and used the natural elements such as air, light, water, food, movement and rest to regain health. Four thousand years before them, Hippocrates, who is known as the Father of modern medicine, underlined two of the main principles of Naturopathy by saying, 'Let food be your medicine and let medicine be your food.' He also emphasized the power of self-healing when he said, 'Only nature heals provided it is given the opportunity.'

Over the last two centuries many of us have lost touch with these ideals as we have become members of an industrialized, urbanized society, with a food and water supply which is increasingly poisoned and polluted. Our diet is far removed from the fresh, more natural raw vegetables, fruits, nuts and seeds, lightly cooked grains and cereals, occasional meat and fish of our ancestors. It is over-refined, is chemically tampered with and, in addition, we eat too much of it! There are signs, however, that people are more aware of the negative effects of such a lifestyle and are looking for alternative methods of combating these problems via the growing demand for organic wholefoods and the support for ecological movements.

PHILOSOPHY

The main principle on which Naturopathy is founded is the same as for other alternative therapies: the importance of the body's natural vitality which leads it towards self-cleansing, self-repairing and self-healing. This mechanism works on its own if nothing is impeding its process.

The body is well equipped to withstand various kinds of internal changes, such as hormonal regulation during the menstrual cycle, and external ones such as the changing seasons. We have an excellent defence system that has evolved over the centuries, but we expose ourselves to all kinds of onslaughts: poor posture and muscle tone due to sitting for too long and lack of exercise, leading to poor circulation and accumulation of wastes; use of drugs which push the symptoms inside and lead to unwanted side-effects; the excessive use of stimuli; occupational hazards such as asbestos dust, VDUs, etc. All these factors and many more break down our defences and lead to disease.

HOW IT WORKS

So what can the body do to deal with all this? It has various ways to free itself of disease and symptoms, the result of which ultimately strengthen the body. Although these can be unpleasant, they are the body's way of re-establishing health and are to be encouraged rather than suppressed. A couple of examples will give you the picture.

First, the body can develop a fever which increases the body's metabolic rate and circulation of blood and lymph, therefore speeding the removal of toxins from the body. A raised temperature also creates a less favourable environment for bacteria. Therefore, in a Naturopathic treatment it is important to let the fever run its course. Secondly, the discomfort experienced in the acute style of a cold is necessary to remove toxins from the body, as irritants, bacteria and viruses stimulate the production of secretions towards the nearest exit. If we do not allow this acute condition to proceed, then waste accumulates within the body and becomes toxic, eventually destroying tissues and organs. This leads to a chronic condition which is harder to treat.

The second principle of Naturopathy concerns the nature of disease, which is the manifestation of the vital force trying to rid the body of any obstructions to its proper functioning. So the Naturopath tries to discover whether the cause is chemical, mechanical or psychological, in so far as we can separate these factors.

A chemical cause of disease would mean an excess of waste products due to poor functioning of the kidneys, lungs and bowels or poor circulation of body fluids such as the lymphatics due to dietary deficiency or dietary excess. A mechanical imbalance can refer to poor posture due to a sedentary occupation. This can lead to a spinal tension which is the malfunctioning of the whole area around the vertebrae so that the nerves, blood supply and the lymphatic circulation are affected. A psychological cause refers to the particular characteristics of the person and how he or she is affected by stress situations in any part of life.

Nothing mentioned so far can take place in isolation, so the Naturopath is concerned with the whole body in its environmental context. The unique response of each individual to that environment is fundamental to the way a Naturopath treats. So the Naturopath takes account of the whole person, trying to find the cause of an illness as opposed to just dealing with symptoms.

WHAT TO EXPECT FROM A VISIT TO A THERAPIST

A standard consultation will take up to one hour and consist of taking a thorough medical history plus questions relating to lifestyle and occupation and, of course, a summary of your diet and eating habits. Other guides to your nutritional status will be used, such as the state of your eyes, hair, skin and nails; if relevant, the Naturopath will take your pulse, blood pressure, check your heart and lungs, and will perform any other basic checks such as examining your eyes or ears. If further tests are needed you will be sent to the appropriate hospital where more specialized equipment is available. This is one of the ways in which alternative and traditional practitioners co-operate with one another.

Most Naturopaths are also Osteopaths and so will examine you structurally by looking at your spine and posture to test the mobility of all the joints and determine whether the nerve and blood supply from the spine are reaching the tissues or organs without being blocked. Possible areas of stress show up when someone has, for example, an excessive curve in the lower back with poor abdominal musculature, which will exert strain on the digestive and pelvic organs.

The Naturopath will be interested in your family history of disease; if such a history exists this will increase your susceptibility to a particular complaint. Your body type will guide the

Naturopath to the kind of diet that will suit you. The soft, rounded endomorph type with large digestive organs, for example, may need a more vegetable-based and fibrous diet which will not putrefy quickly as do animal proteins. Long and lean people – ectomorphs – will want feeding more frequently with more protein.

The kinds of treatment used by a Naturopath are wide-ranging and might consist of one or a combination of the following: fasting and dietary therapy, the structural adjustments of Osteopathy, a relaxing massage, the use of Hydrotherapy (for example, water treatment in the form of packs, compresses or inhalations), exercises (either specific ones for a certain part of the body or general exercise to strengthen, stretch or tone the body, such as swimming or walking), relaxation techniques and, lastly, the common-sense natural hygiene aspect of Naturopathy which looks at how to incorporate a good balance of air, sunlight, movement and water with your lifestyle.

Some form of treatment and advice is given at the consultation; this may include a new dietary regime, some exercises, a relaxation technique to practise or hydrotherapy to do at home. The client always goes away with work to do and will normally return for several follow-up treatments at varying intervals according to the severity and nature of the problem.

How it Fits into an Individual's Lifestyle

Like most alternative therapies, Naturopathy involves taking responsibility for one's own state of health and making changes where necessary with the support of the Naturopath. The client may need to change the balance of his or her life – to take more rest, for example, or more exercise – to make changes to usual dietary habits, perhaps to go on a fast prior to making nutritional changes. It might also involve looking at one's occupation in terms of stress levels. Inevitably, all this involves commitment and finding more time for general health.

Let us take two examples of the range of changes undertaken: first, Client A, coming for treatment for extreme tiredness, an inability to concentrate at work and aching joints. She changed her diet radically after the Naturopath checked her for food allergies. This meant excluding a number of foods and using substitutes (within her already healthy pattern of eating). Together with this she had six sessions of Cranio-Sacral Therapy, a very gentle and effective form of Osteopathy which, with the dietary alterations, lead to a complete restoration of her energies and to pain-free joints.

Client B, on the other hand, has had regular treatment over several years, during which time he has totally reformed his diet, has given up smoking and has had Osteopathic treatment for back pain, old injuries and tension of the diaphragm. He has also worked with meditation and relaxation techniques to help with some of the problems of his past personal life. During this time he has altered his working life from totally manual work interspersed with spells of unemployment to part-time manual work and training as a counsellor. In fact, there was very little in his life that did not alter. On the whole, he has made enormous strides forwards, with only a few steps backward at intervals.

Naturopathy is an active, practically based philosophy, so some adaptations to lifestyle will inevitably be necessary. It is not a soft option, but obviously the Naturopath is there to give positive support, understanding and encouragement. He or she also aims to provide explanations of the processes involved in treatment, so that the client can deal more easily with changes or reactions as they occur. It is not an instant cure: as the examples cited show, treatment may take anything from a few weeks to a few years, and it does involve being prepared to look hard at various aspects of yourself and your life.

HOW IT INTERACTS WITH OTHER THERAPIES

Naturopathy complements many other alternative therapies very well, in that it provides an excellent foundation for good health and gives the individual back the responsibility for his or her own treatment. In addition this foundation can be built upon by using other therapies.

For example, **Herbal Medicine** can be used to strengthen particular systems of the body and to pick up where the Naturopath has left off, if a client has not fully responded to the treatment. I often find the **Alexander Technique** a good complementary therapy to follow on from any osteopathic work which comprises part of a Naturopathic treatment. It can deal with the use of the body in more depth to prevent a recurrence of the problem. Reflex Zone Therapy (known also as **Reflexology)** also works well with Naturopathy. Naturopathic treatment gives the person the building blocks of sound general health, while Reflex Zone Therapy further boosts the inherent healing powers of the body.

Some people find that when working on, say, the physical aspect of their life via Naturopathy, they can successfully pursue the emotional side of things with a psychotherapist **(Psychotherapy).** I find that one feeds and supports the other positively.

Osteopathy and **Massage,** as has already been suggested, form an integral part of the normalizing process and are practised by the majority of Naturopaths. **Acupuncture** and **Homoeopathy** can well be used after getting as sound a basis of health as possible through Naturopathy. Sometimes, given the poor quality of food nowadays, Naturopathy on its own is not enough to restore vital reactions, and for those people who are not ready to go for the level of self-discipline required, the more passive aspects of Homoeopathy or Acupuncture treatment may be more suitable and helpful.

CONDITIONS FOR WHICH IT IS EFFECTIVE

Strictly speaking, Naturopathy treats the person as a whole rather than dealing with specific conditions. However, each of us has different susceptibilities and reactions to exposure to disease. One person will always catch the office cold or flu and have a few days off work, whereas another will have a milder version for two or three weeks, followed by a chronic sinus condition; a third may escape it completely but may be prone to something different, such as stress-related headaches.

There are very few conditions which cannot be treated by Naturopathy, given a commitment to health on the part of the client. As a general rule you can consult a Naturopath about all the complaints you would take to your GP: from coughs, colds, flu, bronchitis, asthma and hay fever to back problems, arthritis, digestive problems (such as colitis or ulcers) and high or low blood pressure. This list is not exhaustive but is meant to give you an idea of the range of possibilities. Like a GP, a Naturopath will send you for further tests if he or she suspects a pathology (an identifiable disease state). You would *not* go to a Naturopath with a fracture, dislocation of a limb, or after an accident where you might need surgery, nor would you go to one if you needed pain relief for a terminal illness, or a life-saving drug following a major heart attack.

QUALIFICATIONS

The Naturopath you will see will have had four years' full-time study at the British College of Naturopathy and Osteopathy (part of the General Council and Register of Naturopaths), where he or she will have studied a range of traditional medical subjects as well as the theory and practice of Naturopathy and Osteopathy. Your practitioner will have needed 'A' levels in Biology and Chemistry in order to do the training.

General Council and Register of Naturopaths
Frazer House
6 Netherall Gardens
London NW3 5RR
Tel. 071 – 435 8728

Incorporated Society of Registered Naturopaths
1 Albemarle Road
The Mount
York YO2 lEN

Further Reading
Beth MacEoin, *Healthy by Nature* (Thorsons, 1994)
Roger Newman Turner, *Naturopathic Medicine* (Thorsons, 1990)

Neuro-linguistic
❧ Programming ❧
JUNI PARKHURST

A Brief History

The first question everyone always asks is, what does Neuro-Linguistic Programming (NLP) actually mean? The 'Neuro' part means that our behaviour comes from our neurological processes of sight, hearing, smell, taste, touch and feeling. We receive information through our senses and form our behaviour accordingly. Mind and body are inseparable and form a recursive system.

The 'Linguistic' part of NLP indicates the verbal and non-verbal language we use to express our individual way of perceiving the world.

The 'Programming' part refers to the ways in which we choose to organize our ideas, experiences and behaviours. Implicit in this idea is that we can choose to 'reprogramme' a behaviour – e.g. a phobia or bad habit, etc. – that has become unsuitable or undesirable.

Origins

NLP was created in the early 1970s and is therefore one of the more modern therapies. Richard Bendler, mathematician and Gestalt therapist, and John Grinder, Professor of Linguistics at Santa Cruz University in the US, together studied brilliant therapists such as Fritz Perls (the originator of Gestalt theory), Virginia Satir (who was an exceptional family therapist) and Milton Erickson (the pioneer of indirect hypnosis). All these therapists had the distinction of being able to achieve improvement or cure with patients who had been written off as beyond help. Bendler and Grinder scientifically studied how these and other therapists achieved results that can only be described as extraordinary. They 'modelled' their way of perceiving the world and their distinctics of thought and behaviour in order to be able to transfer these skills to other therapists.

PHILOSOPHY

NLP has certain central tenets, which are listed below. It is an expanding field, however, and developments are happening all the time as we discover new uses for the skills.

1. The map is not the territory. (We respond to our thoughts and memories. These are our internalized maps of reality. However, these maps are not true reality.)
2. Experience has a structure. When we change the structure, our perception of an experience will change.
3. Mind and body are parts of the same system.
4. We all already have all the resources we need to solve our problems.
5. Memory and imagination use the same circuits and therefore have the same impact, i.e., if something is imagined intensely with all the senses the body acts as though it were real.
6. You cannot not communicate. We are always communicating, even non-verbally. Even thoughts are communication with the self.
7. The person or element with the most flexibility of behaviour in a system has the most influence.

8. There is no such thing as failure; what we may perceive as failure is feedback on how to act and do things differently in future.

WHAT TO EXPECT FROM A VISIT TO THE THERAPIST

Here is an actual account, from the patient's point of view. The patient was a 30-year-old teacher.

I had always had a fear of snakes; I only had to see a picture of a snake on television or in a book to have a panic attack followed by irrational behaviour, involving checking my bed and cupboards to make sure there were no snakes in there. I put off travelling abroad to countries such as Australia, where I had relatives I wanted to see, in case I saw a snake. I had never been bitten or attacked by a snake. The earliest memory I had of seeing a snake was of coming upon one unexpectedly in long grass and the snake winding its way harmlessly away from me, but I felt fear and I suppose the association stuck.

During the session the therapist put me at ease and seemed confident she would be able to help me. I can't say I shared this confidence but I did really want to be free of this phobia. I was asked to visualize myself sitting in a cinema seat looking at an empty screen. When I had achieved this, the therapist touched my arm, telling me this would associate that position with the touch. This was called 'anchoring'. Then I had to see myself sitting in the projection box, looking down at myself, sitting in the cinema still watching the blank screen. This position was 'anchored' in a different place on my arm. I was then guided to remember feeling a pleasant, calm, peaceful state; that state was again 'anchored' separately.

On the cinema screen, from my position in the projection box, I was asked to visualize a still picture of a snake in black and white. I found this distressing and the 'comfort' anchor had to be applied. Slowly I felt better and my panic subsided to the point where I was able to bear the still snake picture.

The 'projection box' anchor was applied, to make sure I was still watching myself watching the screen. Then I was guided to animate the picture, still in black and white, and see my younger self disturbing the snake winding away. I managed that.

Then I had to be in the screen but at the end of the scenario, and imagine that I was being a video wound backwards, very fast and in colour. I did this a couple of times. I then sat in the cinema seat and watched the movie in black and white and then in colour. The therapist asked me to describe my feelings on watching the snake moving and in colour; I could only say that I felt neutral, as though it had all happened a long time ago and it really didn't matter anymore. I opened my eyes and came back to the room.

I was cautiously pleased by this neutral reaction but did not know how I would feel if I saw a snake on television or in a book. Since then I have had the experience of switching on the television at random and seeing a snake on a natural history programme. I felt absolutely nothing except a vague interest in the pattern of its skin and calmly switched to another channel. My family, who had been witness to my panic attacks, are astounded by the change in me and I am delighted, particularly that I can now contemplate travelling to Australia.

HOW IT WORKS

The process the therapist took this client through is called Visual/Kinaesthetic Dissociation; I chose it as a good example to display some of the main features of NLP as used in therapy. (NLP also has wider applications in education, business, consultancy, sports and personal development.)

The therapist worked to change the association of snakes with fear by modifying the sensual intensity of the image, seeing it in black and white (and with the removal of its stripes). The fear was replaced by the neutral feelings so it was impossible to get the old feelings back. NLP is, in short, the study of the process of subjective behaviour. Once an event has happened it cannot be changed – but the perception of the event can be changed.

One of the principal reasons why NLP has become so popular in the US and latterly in the UK is the speed with which such long-standing problems can be solved. The session recounted took one and a quarter hours and the problem had been there 'always'. Many other problems can be solved as quickly.

WHO CAN BENEFIT?

Anyone who has a behaviour that he or she would like to change or improve, e.g. phobias, overeating, smoking, depression, pessimism, post-traumatic stress disorders, allergies, etc., will benefit from NLP. NLP effects improvements in confidence, flexibility, concentration, creativity, memory and decision-making. NLP encourages self-generated change, i.e., patients are not dependent on the practitioner but learn to run their own brain for their benefit. One of the features of NLP which makes it different from other therapies is that it is possible to do 'content-free' therapy. The patient indicates the area of the problem, e.g., phobia, but does not have to describe the problem in detail for the process to be effective.

How it Fits into an Individual's Lifestyle

The sessions last one to one-and-a-half hours and can be taken at weekly or longer intervals to suit the client and therapist.

Goals for Change

The aim of NLP is to make a positive impact on the life of the individual, and changes should be apparent quickly. NLP practitioners believe that transforming debilitating emotions into empowering resourceful states need not necessarily be slow, painful, or based on catharsis. This can therefore mean that you do not necessarily have to go through remembered pain to be free of it. There is a more empowering way of resolving these issues and facing the future. NLP therapy is not a traumatic experience but a positive and self-empowering one.

How it Suits an Individual's Personality

NLP can and does cure problems painlessly and easily. There is also a deeper and more complicated level of NLP, involving modelling of the thought processes of human excellence. This is very popular in the US, where successful business people and sports personalities have been 'modelled' by NLP practitioners, and their positive strategies transferred to others. This is a more protracted process but again leads to excellent results. NLP is a worthwhile therapy for people who value personal power and want to see results quickly, develop their own strategies and not feel over-dependent on a therapist.

How it Interacts with Other Therapies

NLP is a goal- or outcome-oriented therapy as opposed to analysis-oriented, open-ended therapies. In the first session clear criteria are established as to how you (in tandem with the practitioner) will know when you have achieved what you want. This clarification of intention is in itself therapeutic. NLP, perhaps because it is a modern therapy developed within the last 20 years, incorporates an approach where the integrity of the client is respected. The practitioner encourages the client to be the best person that he or she can be, not to fit in with the therapist's ideal of what a 'well-adjusted' person should be. Personal power and autonomy are key issues here. Results and lasting changes should be achieved quickly, and it is considered important to obtain evidence of these results – a goal which, again, is not like those of the longer-term therapies.

NLP can be physical and involve working with body posture. Mind and body are both involved in change. There are certain links with Feldenkrais body work in the sense of working with mind and body as a whole system. NLP can be successfully combined with physical and dietary therapies such as **Herbal Medicine** and body work (**Chiropractic**, **Osteopathy**, etc.).

Qualifications

Qualifications for an NLP practitioner are the same in the UK as in the US. An individual can qualify as a Practitioner, move on to becoming a Master Practitioner and then to becoming a Trainer. These qualifications are internationally recognized through the Society of Neuro-Linguistic Programming (based in the US), and guarantee a level of skill on the part of the practitioner. However, as with any therapy, the client must feel that the therapist is right for him or her. The NLP therapist regards building a rapport with the client as central to the therapeutic process. This does not mean, of course, that the client cannot be challenged, or vice versa, but that the channels of communication between client and practitioner are open.

Association of NLP
48 Corser Street
Old Swinford
Stourbridge
West Midlands PY8 2DQ
Tel. 0384 443935

Further Reading
Joseph O'Connor and John Seymour, *Training with NLP* (Thorsons, 1994)

❧ NUTRITIONAL THERAPY ❧

LINDA LAZARIDES

ORIGINS

Nutritional Therapy is as old as medicine itself. Right up to modern times doctors have always told patients what to eat. It is only since the advent of today's 'wonder-drugs' that nutritional advice is no longer fashionable as a form of medical treatment (with some rare exceptions). Nutritional Therapy really began in earnest in the early days of Naturopathy. Naturopaths such as J. H. Kellogg, Vincent Priessnitz and Sebastian Kneipp in the late 19th/early 20th century used nutrition and fasting, together with other therapies, to cleanse the body and build up its self-healing ability.

Since those days we have learned a lot more about how the body works. We have studied the detailed composition of hormones, enzymes, blood and the intricate workings of the cell itself. We have also learned much more about the composition of food. Vitamins have been identified and studied in minute detail. Essential fatty acids (similar to vitamins) have been discovered. We know how they are broken down (metabolized) and interact with other nutrients to nourish particular body functions. We know how individual amino acids (the building blocks of protein) knit together in enormously complex patterns with other nutrients to produce everything our body consists of.

Specialist practitioners of Nutritional Therapy (at first mainly doctors) began to emerge from the 1950s onwards, using this new knowledge to devise diets and regimes of vitamins and minerals especially targeted at specific symptoms and illnesses. Nutritional

Therapy thus became a much sharper tool, with a scientific basis. This therapy has been developed and fine-tuned over the years, and is now a potentially highly sophisticated health care system which uses a knowledge of physiology and body chemistry to explore all ways of manipulating a patient's nutrition to achieve a desired therapeutic effect. Some of the old Naturopathic principles are incorporated, but generally Nutritional Therapy has developed as a therapy in its own right. Its practitioners have usually been trained at specialist centres (in the UK at least). Some British Naturopaths do incorporate advanced Nutritional Therapy into their treatments, but this depends very much on the individual practitioner.

HOW IT WORKS

A Nutritional Therapist will assess what kind of diet or supplement regime to prescribe, on the basis of the following three broad diagnoses:

1. An allergy or sensitivity to a food or to something in the environment.
2. Toxic overload due to heavy metals or chemicals in the environment, lack of efficiency in eliminating waste products from the body, or poor liver function.
3. Nutritional deficiencies due to poor diet, special needs or malabsorption.

Allergy Diagnosis

A wide variety of problems which can affect the skin, moods, sinuses, digestive system and so on, can be caused by eating something that disagrees with you. This may be a common food such as coffee, bread or sugar. Symptoms may not occur immediately after eating the offending food, but can be delayed, or only appear from time to time – for example when you are stressed.

Toxic Overload

Particularly as age advances, it is possible to have problems due to internal pollution or lack of efficiency in eliminating waste products from the body. These waste products can cause fatigue, fluid retention, arthritis, skin problems and other symptoms as they block and poison body processes.

Nutritional Deficiencies

If your eating habits are not what they should be, or if you are not absorbing all the nutrients from your food, you may have slight deficiencies which could affect your skin, nerves and hormones in particular. It is possible to have symptoms of nutritional deficiency even if you eat a healthy, balanced diet. This is why a Nutritional Therapist often makes use of dietary supplements. Supplements are a minefield for the lay person. Some are made from cheap, poorly absorbed ingredients and are not designed to correct deficiency symptoms. Multivitamin and mineral products may lack a number of nutrients. Nutritional Therapists, on the other hand, have access to special practitioner products designed for safe, expert use.

WHAT TO EXPECT FROM A VISIT TO A THERAPIST

The diagnosis is made primarily by questioning and examining the patient, although some practitioners use methods such as Kinesiology (muscle-testing) or vega-testing (using a machine to

191

measure electrical reactions in the skin). Questions relate to symptoms, medical history, stress factors, lifestyle and eating habits, and the patient may be given a questionnaire to complete which will serve as a basis for discussion and diagnosis. Once the basic diagnosis has been made, the patient is given a treatment regime. The diet prescribed varies according to individual need, and may be a hypoallergenic diet, a cleansing diet, a diet with a high content of specific foods, a diet using a number of foods in rotation, and so on. Supplements used may be vitamins, minerals, amino acids, essential fatty acids, probiotics (beneficial bacteria such as are found in natural yoghurt), enzymes, etc. Some practitioners also use basic herbs and recommend herbal teas.

The initial regime is intended to clear up as many symptoms as quickly as possible, but also to enable the second stage of diagnosis to be reached if necessary. Secondary diagnoses are problems such as adrenal or thyroid exhaustion, liver congestion, candidiasis or malabsorption. They are suggested by the patient's response to the initial regime.

HOW IT FITS INTO AN INDIVIDUAL'S LIFESTYLE

Although the initial diet tends to be restrictive, it does not normally last long. The aim is to fine-tune the diet and supplements gradually, until the least effort, inconvenience and expense on the patient's part are required to maintain the maximum therapeutic effect. This process normally takes about 10 weeks, though the full healing process may take several months longer, depending on the problem. Some patients respond rapidly, but generally a slow, steady improvement is the norm.

Throughout the process, great emphasis is placed on ensuring that the patient can keep to the programme, since there is no point prescribing a diet if a patient cannot stick to it. A good Nutritional Therapist is skilled in helping patients understand how their bodies work, helping them to understand how they can gain control over body functions using the Nutritional Therapy programme, and helping them through any difficulties they might experience.

CONDITIONS FOR WHICH IT IS EFFECTIVE

Nutritional Therapy is all about exploring how an individual's health has gone wrong and helping that individual understand how to put it right using nutrition and knowledge of the body and how to prevent the problem from returning. Practitioners cannot treat every problem with nutrition alone, but of all the therapies this one is the most essential. If your nutrition is not right, other therapies are likely to fail because every part of your body is made from what was once food. Many patients come to Nutritional Therapists after years on Homoeopathy, Acupuncture or other therapies, complaining that these treatments only seemed to work for a limited period – that once the treatment ceased, the problem returned. These patients frequently have a nutritional imbalance of some kind, which other therapies merely helped to alleviate but could not cure.

The problems which most readily respond to Nutritional Therapy used alone are:

Migraine or headaches
Irritable bowel syndrome
High cholesterol levels
Hypertension
Pre-menstrual syndrome
Candidiasis
Overweight

Skin problems
Mood swings of unknown cause
Chronic bloating
Over-acid stomach
Sinusitis
Some types of mental illness
Nausea and vomiting caused by pregnancy

In addition there are a number of illnesses where Nutritional Therapy alone or in combination with other therapies can play an important part in developing the body's strength and resistance, thus helping it to heal itself. Some examples of these are:

Osteoarthritis
Cancers
Rheumatoid arthritis
Heart disease
Diabetes
Multiple sclerosis

How it Interacts with Other Therapies

Most other therapies can be used alongside Nutritional Therapy. Depending on the individual patient and his or her condition, some of the most useful tend to be: **Autogenic Therapy, Hypnotherapy, Osteopathy, Chiropractic** or **Shiatsu**, Lymphatic Drainage Massage (see **Aromatherapy**), Spiritual Healing (see **Psychic Counselling**) and **Bach Flower Remedies**. Most Nutritional Therapists will also advise patients on exercise regimes. For instance, if constipation is a problem, this may be partly due to poor muscle tone in the abdominal area. In overweight patients, an exercise regime may be needed to speed up the patient's metabolism.

FINDING A NUTRITIONAL THERAPIST/QUALIFICATIONS

Finding a Nutritional Therapist may be confusing, since work is only just beginning to organize Nutritional Therapists into a unified profession. Practitioners tend to go under a number of different names, depending on where they trained. The term Nutritionist, Dietary Therapist, Nutritional Therapist, Nutritional Counsellor/Consultant and Clinical Nutritionist encompass those practitioners who specialize in the treatment of allergies, nutritional deficiencies, toxic overload, candida problems, poor digestion, etc. A Mineral Therapist is a practitioner who uses mainly minerals – such as calcium, magnesium and sulphur – but who may add on other forms of nutritional advice. Allergy Therapists and Clinical Ecologists, while similar to Nutritional Therapists, have as their main sphere of action the treatment of allergies and do not always have as much nutritional knowledge. Macrobiotic Counsellors offer an Oriental version of Nutritional Therapy, focusing only on diet, in accordance with the principles of Yin and Yang. Some orthodox medical doctors also offer Nutritional Medicine/Therapy. Unfortunately this does not mean that they are available on the NHS in Britain unless the doctor is listed as a GP.

It is always advisable to find a therapist through a national register; you can find a qualified Nutritional Therapist by contacting the Society for the Promotion of Nutritional Therapy (SPNT), which has a nationwide computerized directory of more than 400 practitioners. It is also involved in educational activities and in unifying the profession. SPNT is working to increase the availability of Nutritional Therapists on the NHS, but this will take many years.

Nutritional Therapists are very different from NHS dietitians, whose work is highly specialized. Dietitians plan diets for the management of patients with liver or kidney disease or diabetes and calorie-counted diets which meet the UK Government's Recommended Daily Allowances for vitamins, minerals and so on. They generally do not work with supplements, the prescribing of which is considered to be the responsibility of the doctors who refer patients to them.

Since all Nutritional Therapy practitioners are very different, before starting treatment it is advisable to ensure that a practitioner is suitable for you by asking for his or her literature and then arranging a short preliminary consultation to ask about the methods used and whether the practitioner thinks they can help you. You should bear in mind that the supplements you will be asked to buy can be quite expensive. However, some practitioners provide treatment at a flat rate which includes all supplements. This usually works out to be a cheaper option.

Society for the Promotion of Nutritional Therapy
First floor
The Enterprise Centre
Station Parade
Eastbourne
East Sussex BN21 1BE
Tel. 0323 430203

Further Reading
Dr Melvyn Werbach, *Healing through Nutrition* (Thorsons, 1994)

❧ POLARITY THERAPY ❧

STEPHAN SCHORR-KON

ORIGINS

Polarity Therapy came out of the lifetime's work and research of Dr Randolph Stone. Dr Stone was Austrian-born but moved to the US as a child in the early years of this century. Although he qualified as a doctor of Chiropractic, Osteopathy, Naturopathy and Neuropathy, he felt that, ultimately, these approaches to healing lacked some vital ingredient. He devoted his early years, during which time he practised and taught medicine in Chicago, to the quest for a unifying principle of medical treatment. His research led him to study traditional systems in the Middle and Far East. He was particularly drawn to the yogic and ayurvedic cosmologies, which gave him the clue to the concept for which he was searching.

What Stone discovered was that all life is energy in motion. This energy, of which each one of us, and all matter, is constituted, arises from a source and returns to it. This insight became the central notion of Polarity Therapy. It led to a whole new perception of the body/mind as an energy matrix.

All life, Stone observed, is movement, and all movement flows from positive through neutral to negative and back again, cyclically. From the same tradition, Stone described energy as having three qualities, or *gunas*: *sattvas* (neutral), *rajas* (positive) and *tamas* (negative). The yogic view postulates a system of chakras or pulsing spheres whose interweaving energy creates the body. In Polarity Therapy these interlinked principles became two of the major reference points for a whole library of significant maps of energy movement in the body. These maps describe a subtle energy network for the geography of being, at the physical, emotional, psychological and spiritual levels.

Initially it is with reference to these maps that the practitioner engages with his or her client on a bodily level. It is an ironic fact that the diagram for these two systems, the *caduceus*, is the symbol of the medical profession, although its meaning has long been forgotten.

HOW IT WORKS

All pain, said Dr Stone, is blocked energy. In Polarity Therapy we trace the movement of energy in the body and seek out the critical blockage or blocked dynamic. Each of the five chakras with which we work embodies an element, and each element resonates at a different frequency: stepping down from ether, through air, fire, water and earth. Each chakra governs a particular organ system, as well as specific ways we relate to ourselves and the world through our emotions and our psychological states. The quality and location of the blockage affecting these elements begins to indicate the nature of the dysfunction the person is presenting. The therapist offers a neutral space in which the client can, through awareness, begin to release contracted energy and regain a balanced energy system, and thus good health.

The practitioner uses four tools in working with clients:

A. Bodywork: the therapist is rigorously trained to listen actively; to feel the qualities of energy and its pulsation; and to look for the whole spectrum of subtle indicators to the client's state. He or she will then work through the body using various levels of touch to connect with, evaluate and move energy in appropriate ways, to dissipate blockages, release contractions and to restore vitality and tone where necessary. As the client's energy system regains balance, health is restored.

B. Presence and contact: the therapist is trained to reflect for the client recurring patterns of unconscious behaviour. Bringing listening and reflecting skills into the therapeutic context allows the client to develop greater awareness of his or her areas of difficulty or dysfunction.

C. Exercises: we employ an array of gentle stretching postures and exercises such as yoga – but again, these will be related to the particular elemental constitution of the client and his or her needs.

D. Diet: the dietary approach looks at the food the client eats and relates that food to its elemental type. A client lacking in fire energy, for example, might need to eat more 'fire foods' (these classifications are explained as we work with clients). We also look at the client's intake of toxins such as drugs, alcohol, tobacco, heavily processed foods and so on. In the case of most chronic illnesses, detoxifying diets are indicated. We also look at the acid/alkaline balance in the client's food. And just as important as the food itself is mindfulness in the preparation and ingestion of food.

Each therapist may bring to his or her practice particular additional skills and training. For example, some practitioners may incorporate Psychotherapy or Herbalism into the practice. It is thus useful to meet the therapist before undertaking a course of sessions.

WHAT TO EXPECT FROM A VISIT TO A THERAPIST

A therapist with one of the qualifications mentioned below would usually use the first session to take a case history. If time allowed or if there were an acute condition, some body work might be done. Unless the client comes in to address a very specific acute dysfunction, a course of possibly six sessions is suggested as a means of exploring blockages or dis-ease in the system. At times a single session can help to resolve an acute condition. In most cases, however, more time is required.

Occasionally the whole process of awareness and self-discovery in itself becomes the aim of the therapy. It can thus develop into a longer journey. Some clients may decide to undergo training to become therapists themselves.

How it Fits into an Individual's Lifestyle

A profoundly important aspect of Polarity Therapy is that it is a co-operative endeavour. The client and therapist work together as a team. The client may be expected to make important changes in lifestyle and diet, to do certain exercises and to incorporate insights that may arise during treatment.

Polarity Therapy is not an instant cure; it will be indicated for anyone who genuinely wants to make changes in his or her life and is prepared to work towards them.

How it Interacts with Other Therapies

Our intention is to work in a way that is complementary to allopathic medicine. With the client's permission, we would seek to consult the client's GP where necessary. Working with other alternative therapies is usually discouraged during the course of treatment, so as to remain clear about the process of change and its attribution. In some cases, however, if the therapist is not trained in a particular field, he or she might refer the client to an appropriate adjunct therapist (for example, a Herbalist).

CONDITIONS FOR WHICH IT IS EFFECTIVE

As Polarity deals with the whole being, and as we perceive all illness to derive from imbalances in the energy system, it is recommended for anyone who is prepared to take responsibility for his or her own health and well-being. Diseases have a pathology. By addressing the energy process that underlies it, the pathology may be arrested or it may be reversed; in cases where it has crystallized to an irreversible degree, we work with the psychological, mental and emotional states that relate to it. By engaging with the subtle energy system we trace imbalances to their elemental source. We encourage the client to retrace the pathological process through to the deepest level of disharmony. Client and therapist then work together to bring the person into a balanced state, in which health is restored.

It follows that any stress-related illnesses are particularly amenable to this treatment. As both illness and health are psychosomatic, this includes a very wide range of applications.

QUALIFICATIONS

There are three Polarity Therapy organizations in the UK and all belong to the British Polarity Council. Those trained by the Polarity Therapy Educational Trust have qualified for the initials RPT (Registered Polarity Therapist). Members of the Polarity

Energetics Practitioners Association use the initials MPEPA. Members of the International Society of Polarity Therapists are designated MISPT. Each Association or Society provides full professional indemnity insurance for its members as well as binding them to professional codes of conduct.

The British Polarity Council is in the process of integrating the qualifying structures in the teaching of Polarity Therapy in the UK with those in the US. The British Polarity Council is a member of the British Complementary Medical Association.

British Complementary Medical Association
Mental Health Unit
St Charles' Hospital
Exmoor Street
London W10 6DZ
Tel. 081–964 1205

Polarity Therapy Association UK
11 Willow Vale
Frome
Somerset BA11 1BG
Tel. 0373 452250

Polarity Therapy Educational Trust
116 Ladysmith Road
Brighton
Sussex BN2 4EG
Tel. 0273 689215

Further Reading
Franklyn Sills, *The Polarity Process* (Element Books, 1988)

❧ PSYCHIC COUNSELLING ❧

ANGELA KIRK

PHILOSOPHY

Psychic Counselling is a way of guiding a person in the search for the true self, so that he or she can reach full potential without limitation. It is both a healing and teaching session, and involves looking into the person's past, assessing the current situation and offering a positive view for the future.

WHO CAN BENEFIT?

Many people choose this sort of therapy because they have found that their lives have become unmanageable, or because they feel isolated and lonely. Others may suffer regular depressions, have addiction problems, relationship difficulties, physical problems such as muscle tension and headaches, or they may feel that their lives lack direction and they need guidance.

The words 'Psychic Counselling' have been chosen because the therapist is using psychic ability both to tune in to the spirit world and to look at the person's aura with clairvoyant sight. From the first visit, the client will experience a spiritual awakening because love and healing energy are channelled through the medium to bring relief from mental stress.

What to Expect from a Visit to a Therapist

Prior to the appointment the therapist will have linked to the spirit world, and will often see the client's loved ones who wish to be remembered and be of assistance. When the client arrives he or she will be asked to choose from among eight coloured cards. The colour chosen enables the therapist to assess how the person is feeling at that particular time. It is only a mood of the moment, but it is very helpful in making a 'spiritual diagnosis'. Later in the session, when the client has relaxed, and with his or her permission, the therapist will look at the aura. The aura is the energy field which surrounds all living things and the colours 'seen' will show the person's physical strength, mental state of health and spiritual awareness. The aura acts as a protection for the physical body and is a visual reflection of the true self.

Our 'true self' is our essential nature, it is who we really are. It includes the ego, with which we normally identify ourselves and from which we create the 'persona' we present to others. The ego is the sum total of all our memories, habits, aversions, opinions and thought patterns and it provides our terms of reference for relating in the world. Understanding the ego is, therefore, a vital tool for self-knowledge. The ego, however, restricts and frustrates us and gives us only a limited perspective on life. The aim of Psychic Counselling is to transcend the ego and become intimate with the self.

Learning about oneself cannot be done with the rational mind. It does, however, require trust so that the person will follow his or her intuition rather than intellect. Many people have difficulty with both trust and intuition, as they are so closely linked with feelings, which can often be suppressed. In order to understand this problem it is necessary to look back at childhood, where learned behaviour may have resulted from conditional love as opposed to unconditional love; the 'legacy' of this in adult life is suppressed feelings.

HOW IT WORKS

Psychic counselling works through the love provided by 'spirit' and by the therapist.

1. To heal the past it is necessary to look at a person's ideas and beliefs about him- or herself. In much the same way that we periodically look through and sort out our wardrobes to clear out unwanted clothes that no longer fit comfortably, it is necessary from time to time to look at our beliefs about ourselves; some of the ideas that we once thought were really good may have come to be too restrictive and rigid.

2. With the pressures of modern living there is often a tendency to control and manipulate life, based on old thinking patterns and learned behaviour, rather than going with the flow which requires trust in one's intuition and in a higher power. Sometimes a crisis occurs due to wrong living and negative thinking, so the therapist will try to help the person to understand him- or herself and to use the technique of creative visualization to promote a positive outlook for the future, thereby following spiritual law, which is perfect.

   To see spiritual law in operation we need only observe nature, where there is an inherent rhythm and flow to life. The tides of the ocean and the rising and setting of the sun follow a pattern; nothing in nature is haphazard. We too have a natural rhythm within ourselves, but this can be upset and our bodies neglected with poor nutrition, lack of exercise, little fun and relaxation and no time for reflection or creativity. With counselling, these areas of life can be explored and people can learn to love themselves and take care of their needs and wants, rather than always striving for success and achievement.

3. When we come to the earth plane as spirits, we adopt the physical body as a vehicle so that we can gain experience in the 'university of life'. It is as if we are actors in a play; if we

make a mistake we simply re-do the scene. When we look back on our lives we will see that we have made mistakes and have subconsciously chosen to 're-do' a similar scenario, again and again until we have dealt with the experience fully. Once we have learned all we can from an event or encounter we can then move forward in the light of experience. These experiences will then show as colours in the aura. So, through life we purify ourselves and raise our vibrations. The best way to achieve this is by meditation – by examining our lives we come to recognize the patterns of our behaviour and thinking – and by connecting with our higher selves for guidance.

4. The spirit world assists our progress whenever we ask for help. We do, however, have free will, so we can only be helped when we ask and seek enlightenment, otherwise the spirit world would be interfering with the law of cause and effect. It was once said that you cannot change the world, but you can change yourself, and by changing yourself you can change the world. By living in the best way we know, we can add to the colours of the aura which is a reflection of our spirituality.

National Federation of Spiritual Healers
Church Street
Sunbury-on-Thames
Middlesex TW16 6RG
Tel. 0932 783164

USA
Common Boundary Inc.
7005 Florida Street
Chevy Chase, MD 20815
Tel. 301–652–9495

Further Reading
Liz Hodgkinson, *Psychic Counselling* (Aquarian, 1994)

❧ PSYCHOTHERAPY ❧

KIRSTI E. HOLM

ORIGINS

Psychotherapy means attending to the mind, the 'psyche' in Greek meaning the mind and 'therapeutikos' meaning to attend or to treat. In the 5th century BC the Greek dramatist Aeschylus wrote of words as 'healers of the sick temper', and through the ages witch doctors, shamans, priests and poets have all in their own way recognized some form of inner world and the unknown powers within every human being. Psychological conflicts have been the source of dramas and poetry for many centuries.

The common ancestor of the Psychotherapist as the term is understood today is Sigmund Freud. His achievement was to be the first person to offer a detailed map of the psyche, to explore the unconscious and its relationship with the conscious mind and to provide a vocabulary for describing psychological processes, developing techniques for revealing the unconscious and tolerating the more damaging results of its conflicts. The idea that psychology offers an explanation for such conditions as hysteria and paralysis was a revelation to Freud, who came from a Germanic tradition of medicine which was firmly embedded in physiology. That our behaviour is somehow influenced by ideas or feelings of which we are totally unaware, is an essential insight to the very heart of Psychotherapy.

Carl Gustav Jung was a Swiss psychiatrist and a close friend of Freud's, and shared many of his ideas. Jung later broke away from Freud completely. This break was mainly the result of Jung no longer being able to accept Freud's excessive emphasis on the important role of sexuality in human development. Jung's thoughts were more optimistic about human nature, more forward-looking than Freud's, and Jung enjoyed working with myths and symbols. It is therefore not surprising that Jungian ideas were taken up by the members of the growth movement and the alternative societies of the 1960s.

In the sixties, the first Centre of the Development of Human Potential evolved on the coast of California. Named after the Esalen tribe of Indians who had bathed in the hot springs there some two hundred years before, a small spa motel opened and came to be used as a weekend retreat and think-tank by such luminaries as Henry Miller, Aldous Huxley and Alan Watts. By 1962 the Esalen Institute had evolved and began to attract humanistic psychology pioneers such as Abraham Maslow, Fritz Perls and Ida Rolf. The Institute became the flagship of the Human Potential Movement, and there Psychotherapy was linked to art, drama and Eastern philosophy and became an instrument for improved self-awareness.

Today, Humanistic Psychotherapy includes many types of therapies such as Gestalt, Primal Therapy, Encounter groups and psychodrama. Techniques often involve working on the body as well as the mind, and some therapies also lay great emphasis on the spiritual side of our nature. From this the term 'holistic' emerged, meaning that the whole person is treated: body and soul (psyche and soma).

PHILOSOPHY

Psychoanalytic methods developed in three stages: first there was the Hypnotic Method developed by Charcot, then the Cathartic Method, which Freud learned from Joseph Breuer and in which the patient was encouraged to talk about the symptoms and their possible cause, and finally, most important of the three, Free Association as developed by Freud. In Free Association the patient lies on a couch and says whatever comes into his or her head. This was the essential step leading to the possibility of looking at true human nature as had never been done before. Through Free Association, Freud aimed to make the unconscious conscious and to discover the links between present symptoms and past experiences. The key is the unconscious mind – that part of the mind whose contents remain almost inaccessible.

Psychoanalysis is termed psychodynamic because of Freud's analogy with physics. Just as dammed up (repressed) water has to find an outlet, repression is the force which originally pushes certain experiences out of consciousness; and it is resistance which keeps them out of consciousness.

Freud was responsible for revealing the significance of sexual drives within every human being. He conceived our motivational drives as forces of energy, fuelling our desires and emotions, conscious and unconscious. He also recognized the existence of other motivational desires such as aggression, but explained that all his patients' conflicts arose over their sexual desires and fantasies; this was the cause of the break with Jung. Certainly the majority of today's psychotherapists have a broader concept of sexuality, and believe that conflicts arise over problems in childhood relationships rather than our suppressed desires for sexual gratification. This belief, however, can lead to disputes regarding the sexual abuse of children, as unfortunately some people still consider sexual abuse to be the child's fantasy and not a reality.

Defence mechanisms are those unconscious processes which help every individual deal with unacceptable aspects of him- or herself, often lying just below consciousness. Repression was the first defence mechanism described by Freud. It is the totally unconscious forcing of unacceptable material back into the unconscious. Other defences include denial projection (externalizing unacceptable feelings and then attributing them to another person – e.g., 'my husband is to blame for everything that is wrong with our marriage'). Reaction formation means going to the opposite extreme to hide unacceptable feelings, for example hate becoming love (husband cannot accept his true feelings of dislike for his wife and becomes totally devoted to her). Another form of defence is the conversion of unacceptable emotions into physical symptoms.

The aim of Psychotherapy is to undo patients' unsatisfactory defences, those of denial or projection, so that the repressed material, feelings and wishes frustrated in earlier life can be revealed and dealt with – thus the energy used to repress gets transformed (see 'The Dynamics of the Personality', below).

Freud presented the concept of total personality, consisting of three major systems:

- ID – the child
- EGO – the I
- SUPEREGO – the 'above I'.

The Id is the impulsive part of us which seeks pleasure and gratification and follows instructual urges regardless of reality or common sense. The Ego is that part of us which is most in touch with the real external world; it represents reason, common sense and the need to behave realistically and coherently. The Superego is the part of us which, through guilt and conscience, criticizes our deficiencies and failure to live up to higher expectations, spurring us to do better. In order to be a mentally healthy person these three systems must form a unified and harmonious organization. If the three systems of the personality are at odds with one another, the person is said to be maladjusted. Such a person is dissatisfied with him- or herself and with the world, and his or her quality of life is reduced.

The Dynamics of the Personality

The form of energy which operates the three systems of personality is called psychic energy; it performs work as does any form of energy. The transformation of bodily energy into psychic energy and of psychic energy into bodily energy is continually taking place, although just how these transformations take place is unknown.

Freud also realized the lasting influence of childhood experiences in peoples' lives. The child may be father of the man, because the child remains in some part of the man's unconscious; therefore in our adult relationships we often repeat our infantile attachments and conflicts. A simple example is the man who marries someone identical to his mother. This tendency to repeat childhood patterns often lies at the root of the patient's problems. Melanie Klein developed these theories of the importance of what she termed 'relationships future'.

Through self-analysis, Freud became interested in the analysis of dreams. He said that dreams are the royal road to the unconscious. Dream analysis is accepted as a major aspect of Psychotherapy.

For Jung, analysis was more a spiritual quest, a religious experience. He saw its aim as being to achieve the integration or wholeness of the personality and to strengthen the psyche so that it could resist future dismemberment. The ultimate goal of psychoanalysis, according to Jung, is Psychosynthesis.

Roberto Assagioli (born in Venice in 1888) describes Psychosynthesis in this way: man possesses a central core of being, a 'self', but for most people this central 'I' is not their true centre. One might say that it is surrounded by a cloud of emotions and desires that whirl around it like the hot gases of a half-formed planet. Man's first task is to recognize his central core and achieve a balance, a position of command, so to speak. The achievement of the sense of Self is the starting point of real development.

According to Jung, the psyche is composed of diversified but interacting systems and levels, and the three levels in the psyche can be distinguished as consciousness, personal unconsciousness and collective unconscious.

Consciousness is the only part of the mind that is known directly by the individual. It appears early in life, probably prior to birth. A child's conscious awareness grows daily through the application of the four mental functions that Jung calls thinking, feeling, sensing and intuiting. In addition to the four mental functions, there are two attitudes that determine the orientation of the conscious mind. These attitudes are extroversion and introversion. The process by which the consciousness of a person becomes individualized or differentiated from other people's is known as individuation. Individuation and consciousness go hand in hand in the development of personality; the beginning of consciousness is also the beginning of individuation.

The *ego* is the name Jung used for organization of the conscious mind; it is composed of conscious perceptions, memories, thoughts and feelings. It plays the vitally important function of gatekeeper to consciousness. Unless the ego acknowledges the presence of an idea, a feeling, a memory or a perception it cannot be brought into awareness. What happens to the experiences that fail to gain recognition by the ego? They do not disappear from the psyche, because nothing that has been experienced ceases to exist. Instead they are stored in what Jung called the personal unconscious. It is the receptacle that contains all those psychic activities and contents which are incongruous with the conscious individuation. They were once-conscious experiences which have been repressed or disregarded for various reasons, such as because they are distressing thoughts, unsolved problems, personal conflicts or uncomfortable moral issues.

The collective unconscious is a reservoir of latent images, usually called primordial images, which refer to the earliest development of the psyche. Man inherits these images from his ancestral past, a past that includes all of his human ancestral past as well as his animal ancestors.

The growth of personality consists of two interwoven structures that make up the total psyche; these structures must be integrated to make a unified whole. The growth process is influenced, either positively or negatively, by a number of conditions including heredity, a child's experiences with his parents, education, religion, society and maturity as a person ages. There is a radical change in development during the middle years of life. This consists of the transition from adapting to the external world to adapting to one's inner being.

Jung believed that dreams are the clearest expression of the unconscious, but he did not believe in using a fixed symbolism or dream book approach, as he felt that much depended upon individual circumstances and the condition of the dreamer's mind. Jung was probably the first person to suggest that in addition to analysing single dreams one could analyse a series of dreams recorded over a period of time.

When a man begins to know himself, to discover the roots of his past in himself, it is a new way of life. The aim of Jungian therapy is to help the individual get in touch with those roots. Analysis is a journey into the crevices of one's mind. Jung said: 'Learn your theory as well as you can but throw it aside when faced with the uniqueness of the human soul,' and today there are almost as many psychotherapies as there are psychotherapists.

WHAT TO EXPECT FROM A VISIT TO A PSYCHOTHERAPIST

While there are many other schools of Psychotherapy, most therapists today are Humanistic psychotherapists. This means that the therapist treats the whole person and not just either the mind or body. They also relate to the person seeking therapy as a human being, rather than presenting themselves as an analyst or technician.

Therapists will refer to 'clients' rather than 'patients', as a patient is someone who is awaiting or undergoing medical care, and they do not view their clients as ill but as individuals who want to improve their awareness and quality of life.

Psychotherapy does not 'do' anything to you, but through a variety of theories and methods helps you understand the vast and complex regions of your mind. It seeks to give you clarity and insight into your own motives and aspirations, enabling you to break out of limiting habits and develop more choice in life. Psychotherapy deals with more deep-seated personal issues than, for example, does Counselling. By taking a person back to childhood and even birth experiences, traumatic events are uncovered, as are life-inhibiting situations.

Most people who are anticipating Psychotherapy want to know how many sessions they might be expected to attend. This is an impossible question to answer because we have to bear in mind that it is the whole person who presents for assistance, not just a set of 'symptoms' and 'aims'. Be prepared to make a commitment to the therapy so that you avoid running away when you encounter difficulties, and be prepared to answer these questions: 'What do I want from the therapy?' and 'How will I know that I have got it?'.

CONDITIONS FOR WHICH IT IS EFFECTIVE

Many people suffer from neurosis in one form or another, ranging from mild discontent, depression, anxiety and/or problems in relating through to crippling disability and unhappiness. Psychotherapy is based on the knowledge that maltreatment of children, as a result of our society's child-rearing and educational practices, causes immense pain. This pain, due to lack of love, care, affection and attention – or as a result of physical or sexual abuse – can rarely be expressed by the child. To do so would be to risk losing the parent's love and sympathy. However, by suppressing these feelings the child slowly kills his or her real self and thereby loses life-force, spontaneity, creativity and the ability to love him- or herself and others. Therapy is a process whereby the lonely suffering child within learns to express and to articulate the suppressed needs, hurts, anger and grief and so regain the freedom to be his or her true self.

Many people who seek Psychotherapy are not necessarily going through a crisis but are looking for ways to improve their relationships and get more out of life. It can also be the starting point for a deeper spiritual journey.

HOW PSYCHOTHERAPY INTERACTS WITH OTHER THERAPIES

The processes of the mind and the body are seen as inter-functioning aspects of therapy. Neurosis is a physiological as well as psychological development: a person literally embodies his or her neurosis. Every emotion, every shock, every frustration has a direct physiological and psychological consequence. Therapies such as **Acupuncture**, **Alexander Technique**, Biodynamic Psycho-therapy, Cranio-Sacral Therapy (see **Cranial Osteopathy**), Rebirthing, Reiki, **Shiatsu**, etc. will work very well in conjunction with Psychotherapy. Hypnosis (see **Hypnotherapy**) is an excellent method of reaching the unconscious mind and therefore naturally goes hand in hand with Psychotherapy.

GLOSSARY

A **psychiatrist** is a medical doctor who specializes in the mind. They primarily treat mental disturbance as a biological malfunction and therefore prescribe drugs as part of treatment.

A **psychologist** is a researcher and scientist who studies human and animal behaviour.

A **clinical psychologist** works specifically within the medical field and is mainly concerned with assessing people for specific treatment.

Psychoanalytic Psychotherapy is a form in which the patient, with the help of the therapist, explores conscious and unconscious thoughts, feelings, and past and present experiences, with the aim of resolving emotional conflicts and personal difficulties.

Psychodrama is a group process. Individuals enact aspects of their life story with the other members, who play the roles of significant others such as father, mother, boss, child, etc.

Psychosynthesis is concerned with the realization of individual potential and, at the same time, avoiding unbalanced growth; its ultimate goal is to harmonize all elements of the personality.

Association of Child Psychotherapists
54 Gayton Road
London NW3
Tel. 071–794 8881

British Association for Counselling
37a Sheep Street
Rugby
Warwickshire CV21 3BX
Tel. 0788 78328/9

Institute of Dream Analysis
8 Willow Road
London NW3 1TJ
Tel. 071–794 8717

The Institute of Family Therapy
43 New Cavendish Street
London W1M 7RG
Tel. 071–935 1651

The Institute of Group Analysis
1 Daleham Gardens
London NW3 5BY
Tel. 071–431 2693

USA
Association for the Development of Social Therapy
c/o Barbara Silverman
474 Third Street
Brooklyn, NY 11215
Tel. 718–499–3759

Further Reading
Susan Quilliam and Ian Grove Stephenson, *Best Counselling Guide*
  (Thorsons, 1991)

❧ REFLEXOLOGY ☙

HELGA TRAMONTIN

ORIGINS

Reflexology is both old and new. Its origins may be traced back to the Chinese, who some 5000 years ago practised a form of treatment using pressure points. Other ancient cultures in Japan, India and Egypt, too, worked on the feet to promote well-being. There is a pictograph of Reflexology being practised which dates from Egypt's 6th Dynasty (around 2330 BC) discovered in the tomb of Ankhmahor – known as the Physician's Tomb – at Saqqara. Evidence has also been found which suggests that Native Americans and some tribes of Africa employed some form of Reflexology.

In the early years of the 20th century Dr William Fitzgerald, an American physician and surgeon from Connecticut who also worked at hospitals in London and Vienna, systematized the body into zones; the treatment which emerged from his research was later known as Zone Therapy. One of the students of Zone Therapy was Eunice Ingham, a Physiotherapist. She argued that since the zones ran through the entire body, it would make sense to target the feet for treatment as they were more accessible and very sensitive. Eunice Ingham should be credited with being the first person to separate the practice of working foot reflex areas from Zone Therapy in general. She charted the body onto the feet, and thus the maps for modern Reflexology evolved. Doreen Bayly, a student of Eunice Ingham, introduced Reflexology to Britain in the early part of the 1960s.

PHILOSOPHY

The goal of Reflexology is the restoration of a state of equilibrium or balance. If a person is to be healthy, all systems of the body must work together in harmony. If any part is out of alignment, other parts suffer as a consequence. The feet have a special relationship with the body: there are 7,200 nerve endings present in the feet that interconnect with every part of the body. By applying a specific pressure massage it is possible to trigger the body to correct imbalances, to stimulate or calm underactive or over-active areas respectively, to cleanse and to revitalize.

HOW IT WORKS

Reflexology is based on the theory that the body is divided into 10 longitudinal zones: five on each side of a median line through the body. Each zone relates to one of the digits on each side of the body:

> Zone one extends from the thumb up the arm to the brain and then down to the big toe
> Zone two extends from the second finger, up the arm to the brain and then down to the second toe
> Zones three, four and five extend similarly from the third, fourth and fifth fingers to the corresponding toes on each side of the body.

These longitudinal zones are of equal width and extend right through the body from front to back. All organs and parts of the body lie along one or more of these zones. Working any zone in the foot affects the entire zone throughout the body.

In addition to these 10 zones, there exist in the body three transverse zones which can be marked on the body by drawing three lines as follows: across the shoulder girdle, across the waist and across the pelvic floor. These areas can be transposed onto the feet. The longitudinal and transverse zones together form a grid within which the reflex areas can be located.

Hand Reflexology

Reflex areas corresponding to all the parts of the body are also found in the hands. They are similarly arranged to those in the feet, but as the hands are smaller than the feet, reflex areas here are correspondingly smaller and a little more difficult to determine precisely. They also tend to be less sensitive. However, in cases where treatment of a foot or both feet is not possible due to infection or injury, the hand or hands may be treated instead.

The Basic Technique

In general the therapist uses his or her thumb to apply pressure to the reflex areas. The thumb (right or left) is held bent, and the side and end of the thumb are pressed firmly onto each reflex point. On some areas it may be more convenient to use another finger or fingers to apply the compression massage. The therapist's hands carry out complementary functions during treatment, one working and the other supporting.

WHAT TO EXPECT FROM A VISIT TO A THERAPIST

Reflexology is a holistic therapy and seeks to treat not only symptoms but the causes of symptoms. It activates the self-healing mechanism of the body, but the speed with which the healing occurs varies from individual to individual. Often an improvement is brought about after one or two sessions. Chronic complaints, however, take longer to correct. Factors such as diet, lifestyle and attitude play an important part in the healing process, and the co-operation of the patient is invaluable. Once responsibility for his or her own state of health has been accepted, the body will respond more rapidly.

If a specific complaint or complaints are to be addressed, a treatment once a week would be indicated. The sessions can then be spaced out to every other week and later to monthly visits until the condition has cleared up satisfactorily. Visits to a Reflexologist for a 'tune-up', for example once a month, are an excellent way of strengthening and balancing the energy flow and can eliminate potential problems in their initial stages.

What Happens on a First Visit

On a first visit to a Reflexologist a medical history will be taken. Any major illnesses and operations should be mentioned, as well as any medication being taken or any other treatment being administered. The patient will then remove shoes and socks or stockings and recline on an adjustable couch, knees slightly elevated by a wedge-shaped support cushion. The practitioner will then proceed with an examination of the feet. The practitioner will note their colour, temperature, any excessive perspiration, tissue and muscle tone, the presence of hard skin, any corns, verrucas, scars or injuries, as well as any swelling, puffiness or the presence of an infection such as athlete's foot.

A gentle massage with some talcum powder follows, which prepares the feet for the treatment and allows the patient to get used to the therapist's touch. The actual treatment takes about 50 minutes. At the end of it the feet will be given some gentle manipulation; the session concludes with a breathing exercise, leaving the patient relaxed and tranquil.

What a Reflexology Treatment Feels Like

Patients who are new to Reflexology are sometimes tense and apprehensive before a first appointment. Treatment should never be too uncomfortable, as the practitioner will always adjust the amount of pressure applied to suit each individual. Some people are embarrassed about their feet and unused to having them touched. To the trained Reflexologist they represent a map of the body, and each part of them is capable of telling a unique and interesting story. Occasionally patients will worry about having a treatment because their feet are very ticklish. Since the pressure is precisely targeted on the reflex points and is firm rather than tentative, this problem does not really arise.

No two people react in precisely the same way to a treatment. Sensations vary on different parts of the feet and can range from a feeling of something sharp being pressed into the foot to a dull ache, tightness or simply pressure. The sensitivity experienced varies not only from person to person but also from treatment to treatment in the same individual, depending on a number of factors such as stress, mood, time of the day and the state of health at that moment.

Tender reflexes are not necessarily indicative of poor health, nor are insensitive reflexes always a sign of good health. As a rule, however, pain will occur in areas where energy blockages are present. As treatment progresses the reflex areas become less sensitive. Most patients experience a sense of deep relaxation and tranquillity throughout the treatment and find the touch of the Reflexologist comforting and reassuring. On completion of the session the majority feel calm, energized and rejuvenated. Occasionally people report feeling fatigued, especially if they were exceptionally tired to begin with.

Possible Reactions to Treatment

Increased urination
Increased activity of the bowels
Increased secretions from mucous membranes resulting in
   coughing with phlegm and sneezing
Increased discharge from the vagina
Increased perspiration and aggravated skin conditions
Change of sleep patterns – deeper or more disturbed sleep
   may result
Tiredness

All these reactions can be considered positive ones. They form part of the healing process and are of short duration.

CONDITIONS FOR WHICH IT IS EFFECTIVE

Reflexology is very effective in overcoming or alleviating a wide range of complaints, but it is also much more than a remedial treatment to be applied only when ill. People who enjoy general good health but who have to face some or all of the following problems as they go about their work will benefit:

Tiredness and irritability
Aches and pains due to a sedentary occupation
A weak immune system
Stress
Difficulty in building up depleted energy reserves
Travel fatigue and jet-lag

WHO CAN BENEFIT?

Reflexology is a very gentle but powerful and effective therapy. Diagnosis and treatment are totally natural procedures, involving no drugs or instruments. It co-exists happily with other therapies; in fact, practitioners of other complementary therapies often use it as a diagnostic tool before following on with their own forms of treatment.

It is equally important for busy and active men and women to take advantage of a therapy which ensures that the body will function harmoniously and efficiently by instilling deep relaxation and an incredible sense of well-being. Anyone can enjoy the benefits of Reflexology – a therapy which suits all lifestyles.

QUALIFICATIONS

Although the method of treatment may sound quite simple, it is advisable to consult a qualified practitioner. A professional treatment involves much more than the ability to locate the reflex areas. A thorough knowledge, not only of the direct but also of the associated reflexes which need to be worked for specific disorders, is required.

There are a number of conditions where Reflexology treatment could be contra-indicated, and some where extra care needs to be taken, including cases where patients are on specific medication.

It is best to contact a practitioner who is a member of a professional association. Reflexology is today practised in many countries. The legal requirements for qualification differ from country to country or, as in the case of the US, from state to state and, indeed, from city to city.

Association of Reflexologists
110 John Silkin Lane
London SE8 5BE

The British Reflexology Association
Monk's Orchard
Whitbourne
Worcester WR6 5RB
Tel. 0886 21207

Institute for Complementary Medicine
PO Box 194
London SE16 1QZ
Tel. 071–237 5165

International Federation of Reflexology
51 Champion Close
Croydon
Surrey CR0 5SN
Tel. 081–680 9631

International Institute of Reflexology
Francis Wagg, UK Director
15 Hatfield Close
Tonbridge
Kent TN10 4JP
Tel. 0732 350629

Further Reading
Avi Grinberg, *Holistic Reflexology* (Thorsons, 1989)
Nicola M. Hall, *Thorsons Introductory Guide to Reflexology* (Thorsons, 1991)
Nicola M. Hall is Chair of the British Reflexology Association and Director of The Bayly School of Reflexology.

Kevin Kunz and Barbara Kunz, *The Complete Guide to Foot Reflexology* (Thorsons, 1984)

Franz Wagner, *Reflex Zone Massage* (Thorsons, 1987)

❧ RELAXATION MASSAGE ❧

KARIN WEISENSEL

ORIGINS

Massage is probably one of the oldest forms of healing and has been used widely throughout history. The earliest mention of massage appears in a Chinese book dating back more than 2000 years BC:

> *Early morning stroking with the palm of the hand, after the night's sleep, when the blood is rested and the tempers relaxed, protects against colds, keeps the organs supple and prevents minor ailments.*

Numerous references to massage are also found in Greek and Roman literature. Galen, one of the greatest physicians and anatomists of antiquity, wrote several books relating to massage and described the massage given to the gladiators before and after a fight.

In India massage is also greatly valued as part of ayurvedic medicine, and mothers still massage their babies the same way as they probably did hundreds of years ago. However, it was not until the beginning of the 19th century that the therapeutic value of massage began to be recognized and developed throughout the Western world. In 1820 Henrik Ling established the first school offering massage, in his native Sweden. He combined his experience of massage and exercises, gained from extensive travel to various countries and knowledge of diverse cultures, to develop the technique now known as Swedish Massage. Swedish Massage, like most Western massages, is restricted to working only with muscles and soft tissue. The aim of holistic or therapeutic massage, on the other hand, is to treat the whole person, body, mind and spirit. Naturally the basis of all massage, whether Swedish, holistic or any other form, according to various schools of thought, is touch.

HOW IT WORKS

To touch and be touched is an instinctive need in all of us. In daily life we take in information using our eyes to see, our ears to hear, our noses to smell, our mouths to taste and last, but not least, our body to feel. For most people the visual and auditory inputs are the primary sources of information, constantly analysing and responding to given information and leaving little time to experience how we feel, to touch and be touched.

Of all the senses, touch is the first one to develop, and if a person is deprived of touch he or she can feel lonely, depressed and isolated. Touch means contact – contact with others but, most importantly, contact with ourselves. Massage can allow you to get in touch with the most inner core of your being and can help you to become more conscious of your body as a whole. It can therefore be a very emotional and powerful experience.

To make a massage work, both participants must shift their awareness from a visual or auditory mode to a feeling mode and prepare a mental space for the massage to happen. Massage is a two-way process of touch. The hands of the giver and the skin of the receiver work together. Often, no more than a caring touch is needed to melt the armour of everyday stress.

Massage is usually performed on a table with the use of oils, which can be scented, to lubricate the skin and allow the hands to slide smoothly over the outlines of the receiver's body without friction. Stress is the body's worst enemy and we, in our Western society, need to learn to have breaks. Often our bodies no longer even know how to take a break and have become like 'a brick wall with a bank account'. Massage can help to release or soften this 'brick wall', these tensions, aches and pains accumulated in daily life.

WHO CAN BENEFIT?

By stretching and toning the muscular tissue, massage helps to eliminate toxins, encourage the lymphatic flow and stimulate the circulatory system. It soothes our nerves and produces a state of relaxation and well-being. Conditions such as back pain, headache and insomnia are the most common for which someone seeks the help of a Massage Practitioner. Studies have shown that more and more GPs now recognize the benefits of massage and suggest treatments instead of prescribing drugs. However, whether you have a massage to deal with a health complaint or just to unwind from the hustle and bustle of everyday life, it will truly be a memorable and enjoyable experience.

The Association of Massage Practitioners
Flat 3
52 Redcliffe Square
London SW10 9HQ
Tel. 071–373 4697

Australia
Association of Massage Therapists
19a Spit Road
Mosman NSW 2088
Tel. 969 8445

Further Reading
Nigel Dawes and Fiona Harrold, *Massage Cures* (Thorsons, 1990)

Gordon Inkeles, *New Massage* (Thorsons, 1985)
Gordon Inkeles and Murray Todris, *The Art of Sensual Massage* (Thorsons, 1992)

❧ REMEDIAL MASSAGE ❧

JOHN VON HOFF

ORIGINS

Massage Therapy can, in very general terms, be divided into two types: relaxation and remedial. The purpose of Remedial Massage is, as the name implies, to afford a remedy for both specific complaints and ailments and to relieve the deep-rooted stresses and tensions of life today. The Remedial approach to massage, which by necessity uses deeper and more penetrating techniques, is very popular in the Far East where there is a long-standing tradition of serious 'body work' which concentrates more on the patient's health and well-being than might be the case with more superficial Western relaxation techniques.

In the early 5th century BC, Hippocrates, the 'father of medicine' wrote,

> *The physician must be experienced in many things...but assuredly*
> *in rubbing, for rubbing can bind a joint that is too loose, and loose*
> *a joint that is too rigid.*

Bearing in mind that the muscular system is really dependent upon active exercise for its well-being, Remedial Massage can be invaluable in maintaining reasonable muscle tone for those persons who find themselves with limited time to exercise, or who, by their occupation, develop bad posture.

How it Works

Working muscles produce waste products which can cause stiffness when these muscles are subsequently resting. By the regular use of Remedial Massage one can, however, stimulate the blood supply to the muscles and thereby increase the amount of oxygen they receive. This, combined with accelerated lymphatic circulation, will absorb the accumulated toxins and remove any discomfort felt.

Conditions for Which it is Effective

Stress-related aches and pains due to chronic muscular stiffness and strain commonly occur around the lower lumbar region, the upper back, along the tops of the shoulders and the back of the neck. Severe lower back pain may become 'referred' to parts of the legs. Muscular tension is a prime cause of fatigue and may in addition lead to insomnia or disturbed sleep. Faulty posture also creates muscular strain and pressure on nerve centres, thereby contributing to chronic ailments such as migraine, headaches and back pain. Sedentary occupations coupled with lack of exercise encourage obesity, placing stress on the heart and lungs, weakening muscles and stiffening the joints. Symptoms such as frozen shoulder, tennis elbow and other similar complaints can often be greatly relieved by Remedial Massage, as can problems with ligaments and tendons.

A very important additional form of remedial therapy is the use of Cranial Massage. Headaches and migraine are commonly early warning signs of excessive stress, which manifests itself as muscular tension. Involuntary grinding of the teeth or clenching of the jaw and the tensing and tightening of facial muscles may lead to other forms of stress-related facial pain such as neuralgia. Persons suffering from these symptoms will often obtain tremendous relief by having specific Cranial Massage Therapy.

How it Interacts with Other Therapies

Other therapies such as **Chiropractic**, **Osteopathy** and **Alexander Technique** are more easily performed on patients whose muscles are properly relaxed, and to this end Remedial Massage proves particularly useful as a preparatory therapy. Patients who have experienced Remedial Massage tend to feel a deep sense of well-being; they feel relaxed, loose and comfortable. Their work, sleep and eating habits all improve and their increased energy gives them the ability to cope more readily with all the everyday stresses and tensions.

Association of Massage Practitioners
Flat 3
52 Redcliffe Square
London SW10 9HQ
Tel. 071–373 4697

Australia
Association of Remedial Masseurs
22 Stuart Street
Ryde NSW 2112
Tel. 878 2159

✥ ROLFING ✥

LOAN TRAN

Rolfing is designed to realign and restore balance to the body's structure and movement. It does this by manipulation of the connective tissue system: the principal parts on which Rolfing works are tendons, ligaments and the muscular wrappings called the *fascia*. Movement education is also a key element in Rolfing.

ORIGINS

The technique was developed by Dr Ida P. Rolf (1896–1979), an American biochemist who took her PhD in Biochemistry from the College of Physicians and Surgeons of Columbia University. She also studied Osteopathy, Yoga and Homoeopathy, all of which contributed to the development of what she called 'Structural Integration' and which became known as 'Rolfing'. A practitioner of Structural Integration is known as a 'Rolfer'.

Dr Rolf, like many pioneers of new health techniques, developed her method to meet practical needs. One of her sons suffered from poor health which orthodox medicine was unable to improve and doctors had told her that she herself had spinal arthritis which would confine her to a wheelchair. Unsatisfied with the treatment available she travelled around the world researching different approaches to promoting health. Rolfing grew out of her observations and her knowledge of biochemistry. As a result, her son's health improved and she was able to teach until she was well into her eighties.

She first taught her format of 10 Rolfing sessions in Tunbridge Wells in the 1950s, and went on to teach in the US and Canada as well as often returning to Britain. She established the Rolf Institute in Boulder, Colorado in 1973 to train teachers to continue her work.

One of the premises in Yoga which particularly attracted Dr Rolf is that a better balanced body enhances not just the physical but the overall well-being of a person. This premise is also a cornerstone of Rolfing, and people who have been Rolfed often report not just physical improvements but positive changes in many different aspects of their lives.

PHILOSOPHY

The basic principles of Rolfing could be summed up as follows:

Structure and Function are Interdependent

In other words, the way we are built or the way we move influence each other. For example, if you have ever had the bad luck to pick a supermarket trolley which had a wheel that turned outwards you will know how much effort it takes to push the trolley in a straight line. Accordingly, if one of your feet is rotated outwards, the rest of your body will find it that much harder to move straight ahead (try it – you'll find that the foot that turns out will pull that side of your body to one side, and that moving straight forward takes a lot of effort).

Our Bodies and the Way We Move are Subject to the Force of Gravity

We tend to forget that gravity is a constant physical force which affects us. We carry the weight of our bodies under this force; if our bodies are organized so that the different segments can be supported and aligned in harmony with gravity, our posture and movement can be much more easy. Have you ever tried to carry a stack of books which weren't placed in a straight column? When the body is poorly aligned gravity cannot flow through easily. The body is pulled down and it has to work hard to keep itself balanced.

The Whole Body Operates as a System

Structural imbalance in one part of the body leads to compensations in another. For example, if you have ever fallen you know how different parts of your body reacted. Your hands went out to try and break the fall, perhaps you stiffened your neck in fright and so on. If we look at the body as an interrelating structure we see that working on isolated problem areas does not lead to sustained improvement. If you do not address the whole system the compensations will pull structures back out of line and the same problems will recur.

Thus, Rolfing is offered as a series of sessions (normally 10), which can be followed by top-up sessions. Each session addresses certain areas of the body and the series follows a logical progression designed to take the body through a gradual process of realignment and re-education. Each session lasts for between and hour and an hour and a half.

CONDITIONS FOR WHICH IT IS EFFECTIVE

The technique can be effective for dealing with chronic structural problems, lower back pain, stiff neck and shoulders, weak knees, etc. which have not improved with isolated, local treatment. Like Homoeopathy, Rolfing does not try to cure symptoms but rather, as Dr Rolf put it,

We are interested in making a more adequate body for men and women so they can disregard the problems of the body and stick to the things they want to stick to – their job or their sports. We don't set out to 'cure' a body. But we get that body to grow to a place of greater strength and adaptability, greater grace in movement and greater capacity for moving and adjusting.

Dancers, sports people, musicians and other performers who need their bodies to be in optimum condition often use Rolfing to enhance their performance. Rolfers have worked with top-class sports people to help them increase their physical capabilities.

What to Expect from a Visit to a Rolfer

At the first appointment the Rolfer takes time to ask the client's medical history, particularly to find out if there have been any operations or broken bones. Areas which have suffered shock or trauma can be sensitive and when they are touched there can be an emotional as well as physical response.

The Rolfer works with his or her hands to reorganize the connective tissues and release areas which may have become stuck as a response to injuries or movement habits. The client is encouraged to develop sensory awareness and often a technique known as 'comparison' is used to stimulate this. For example, the first session is aimed at freeing restrictions so that breathing can be fuller. First of all one side of the chest and shoulders is worked with and, before continuing to work with the rest of the body, the Rolfer will ask the client to feel if there is a difference between the two sides. The client often notices that his or her breathing is more expansive and that he or she feels more fullness and depth in the chest on the side that has been Rolfed. The client is also expected to participate and assist the manipulations by following precise movement and breathing cues.

The client and Rolfer work together, looking at the client's posture and basic movements such as standing, walking and sitting. Together they identify muscular restrictions and explore more graceful and economical ways of moving, suited to each person as an individual. The Rolfer does not attempt to impose new ideals which could create new tensions as the client strains to imitate or reproduce a standard ideal (there's nothing like someone telling you to stand up straight to immediately make you feel stiff!).

HOW IT FITS INTO AN INDIVIDUAL'S LIFESTYLE

The intervals between sessions can range from one week to a month; each individual is encouraged to find the rhythm which suits him or her best. There can be a deep release of tension during sessions. Sometimes clients make psychological connections to certain physical reactions. For example, working on an area which has been injured may evoke memories of the accident that led to the injury and there may be an emotional response. The Rolfer is prepared for this and provides a therapeutic and safe environment so that the client feels supported. Often clients try to schedule some time alone to themselves afterwards so that they can fully benefit from this relaxation, taking time out to 'bask' in the positive after-effects of Rolfing treatment.

One or just a few sessions can be enough to relax and give an improved sense of alignment. However, the basic series of 10 has been developed to accompany the person through a gradual process so that the benefits are deeper and more sustained. Clients often feel that once their bodies have the sensation of better alignment and balance, old habits no longer feel comfortable. Often they resume or begin a physical activity because they feel an improvement and want actively to maintain this sense of well-being.

HOW IT INTERACTS WITH OTHER THERAPIES

Rolfing can be complementary to other structural therapies such as **Osteopathy** and **Chiropractic**. These techniques can be extremely effective in cases of recent or localized injury, and Rolfing supports the work done with the local problem by encouraging the whole of the body to be in balance. Bones are part of the connective tissue system and, by working with the soft tissue surrounding and interpenetrating the bones, Rolfing helps to sustain the improved alignment that results from osteopathic and chiropractic manipulations.

It can also be an effective adjunct to **Psychotherapy**. Clients who are already in Psychotherapy sometimes want a physical dimension to their therapeutic process. Rolfing, like Psychotherapy, aims to integrate body and mind. For example, Rolfing is not a matter of doing away with a bad knee but evoking better balance so that it can move more appropriately. Likewise, Psychotherapy does not try to eliminate difficult or painful feelings by suppressing them but helps the person to integrate them so that they are not so debilitating. Thus these two approaches help different, and often conflicting, physical and psychological parts to be better integrated. Sometimes clients decide to begin Psychotherapy during (or after) Rolfing, as their increased awareness evokes a desire for change in other areas of their lives. As mentioned, Ida Rolf's attitude was that her technique should be life-enhancing, affecting the whole person – not just a quick fix-it.

QUALIFICATIONS

The selection process for Rolfing training is rigorous; one prerequisite is that candidates have therapeutic experience so that they can work sensitively and empathically with their clients.

The Rolf Institute world headquarters is located in Boulder, Colorado; the European central office is in Munich. Its teaching faculty travels all around the world making the training available in the US, the Pacific Basin, Brazil and Europe. There is continuous research to keep the training up to date with the latest developments in working on the body. Rolfers are also required to follow a continuing education programme which ensures they continue to add to their skills. Irrespective of where they have trained, the Rolf Institute Diploma qualifies Rolfers to work anywhere in the world. It provides a solid basis which individual Rolfers can then adapt to suit the needs of any culture they choose to work with.

European Rolfing Association
Ohmstrasse 9
80802 Munich
Germany

Rolf Institute Headquarters
205 Canyon Boulevard
Boulder, CO 80302
USA

❧ ROSEN METHOD BODYWORK ❧

ULRIKA THAM

ORIGINS

Marion Rosen developed her method from 50 years' experience as a physical therapist and health educator. Her own approach to bodywork has earned her recognition as a leader in the field of body-oriented therapies, principally in the US and Scandinavia. Her own training began in Munich in the 1930s. She trained with Lucy Heyer for two years. Lucy Heyer was the wife of Dr Gustav Heyer (a colleague and former student of Carl Jung). They were part of a group of people using massage, breathwork and relaxation in conjunction with psychoanalysis. This was the beginning of Marion's understanding of the connection between mind and body. She then trained as a physiotherapist in Sweden and later in the US, where she has worked for over 40 years.

PHILOSOPHY

The Rosen Method is based on the premise that there is at one's core a true authentic self. Through social conditioning one becomes increasingly out of touch with this self, living and acting largely unconsciously through a system of masks and self-protecting pretences. During the process of socialization, mental and emotional contractions, the result of fearful experiences which were too painful to manage at the time, are stored in the body in the form of chronic muscular tension. For example, a baby has no trouble expressing feelings spontaneously, usually by crying, yet as this baby grows he or she becomes aware that crying is not permitted or valued as a means of expression. When tears come, the child stops them by tightening the muscles of the neck and chest. When the urge to cry comes again, the child tightens the muscles of the neck and chest and refrains from crying. Later on, the tightening of the neck and chest muscles becomes habitual and the child no longer experiences even the urge to cry. Thus repression is complete and the child grows into an adult with a chronically stiff neck and non-moveable chest and shoulders.

To quote from Marion Rosen,

If you do not let yourself be the way you are, your body cannot function. The same is true for the emotions. The only way you can be who you are is through surrender and self-acceptance.

HOW IT WORKS

The Rosen Method is a gentle hands-on approach to bodywork. Working with those muscles which have been contracted, the practitioner seeks to bring about the client's physical and emotional awareness through relaxation.

Usually the touch in this work is light and soft. Sometimes pressure is used, but never force. As the muscles relax and the breath deepens, feelings, attitudes and memories held in the body begin to surface. Sometimes there is a need to talk about what is happening, sometimes there are tears, and sometimes a deep relaxation is experienced. Often at some later time forgotten memories surface, or dreams become more vivid. The practitioner's key to unlocking the client's habitual holding is the breath. He or she focuses on subtle changes in the breathing as a guide to what is happening in the client's inner process. The practitioner also learns to listen through the hands. The shape of the body, its muscular holdings, tensions and the pattern of the breathing all have their stories to tell and contribute to make the overall picture of whom we are pretending to be, whom we fear we might be and who we really are.

The Rosen Practitioner is not there to fix anything, but simply to draw attention to where there is a holding back and where the client is denying his or her true self. He or she does this by drawing awareness to the physical tension, meeting the barrier with his or her hands and asking the client to talk about the experience of it. Again, it is the quality of consciousness and focus that the practitioner brings to his or her hands that creates the safe environment in which old painful thoughts and emotions can be evaluated. The very fact that these old hurts are stored in the body means that they are buried deep in the unconscious mind and may not be easily explained. The breath is seen as the interface between the conscious and unconscious systems. Through the breath we begin to have access to emotions, feelings and experiences which were previously put away or repressed. As the client's muscular tension relaxes, the physical and emotional barriers which have developed begin to dissolve and the client experiences a new sense of health and well-being.

Marion Rosen states:

> This work is about transformation from the person we think we are to the person we really are. In the end, we cannot be anyone else.
>
> What is in your body is in your unconscious. If you think you know what it is, that is not what it is. The holding is an unconscious holding. You cannot tell the story. The story you can tell is made up of what you have already handled. Pain is a guide to the surfacing of what is unconscious, something repressed. The real pattern is in your unconscious and it has not surfaced yet. When it surfaces, it often takes care of the pain. Very often the

pain disappears in the course of handling whatever the emotion was.

WHAT TO EXPECT FROM A VISIT TO A THERAPIST

A session lasts for one hour. During the first session there is a short interview to ascertain whether the therapy is suitable. The work aims to bring about deep relaxation, so tiredness is a very common after-effect. For this reason it is advisable to book sessions for whatever part of the day which will allow you time afterwards to reap the full benefits.

HOW IT FITS INTO AN INDIVIDUAL'S LIFESTYLE

As the Rosen Method is an inner process it is important to make space and time for yourself, and to be open to changes in your life. It is of value to have a 'supportive environment' either from family or friends, as feelings of vulnerability or deep pain may surface and can be difficult to handle.

HOW IT INTERACTS WITH OTHER THERAPIES

It is important to state that the Rosen Method is not Psychotherapy, although it does work very well in conjunction with **Psychotherapy**. Sometimes Psychotherapy is recommended during the process if too many feelings surface for the client to handle on his or her own.

Generally speaking there are no obvious problems associated with combining the Rosen Method with other therapies.

HOW IT SUITS AN INDIVIDUAL'S PERSONALITY

This method is not an instant cure, but there are documented case histories of a single session resulting in the release of a traumatic event and the disappearance of all pain, after which no further sessions are required. However, the Rosen Method is more often a long-term therapy that requires a commitment on the part of the client to getting in touch with repressed feelings and chronic muscle tension, and taking responsibility for him- or herself. Treatment is recommended once a week or every other week, if possible.

CONDITIONS FOR WHICH IT IS EFFECTIVE

Rosen Method Bodywork is effective for stress-related problems such as backaches and headaches which do not respond to other treatments, and generally problems that fail to respond to more orthodox methods.

It is not suitable for people with depression, those who are taking antidepressants or tranquillizers or for people who are mentally unstable. You need not have a particular ailment to benefit from this method. It is more an exploration into the self, to live a fuller life with greater awareness and more choices in your actions.

QUALIFICATIONS

The training for a Rosen Method practitioner is of three years' duration and at present is available only in the US and Scandinavia. Many of the therapists have other qualifications, such as in Psychotherapy, physiotherapy or other bodywork, but this is not a requirement.

❧ Shen Tao Acupressure ❧

Clare Walsh

Origins and Philosophy

Shen Tao (meaning 'Spirit Path') is a form of vibrational healing which has its origins in the philosophical and medical traditions of ancient China. It was developed in Britain in the mid-1980s by Eliana Harvey, an accomplished healer, together with other members of the Shen Tao Foundation.

As a therapy it is renowned for its gentleness, subtlety and power, and for its ability to release and transform old patterns and habits in a compassionate way which involves a minimum of suffering for the patient.

It is sometimes described as 'acupuncture without needles'; light finger contact is used on specific acupuncture points on the body, in particular sequences with the purpose of rebalancing the patient's vital energy at a profound level.

How it Works

The practice of touching specific points on the body to promote well-being is said to have originated in China several thousand years ago; by the time the earliest Chinese medical text had been written (in about 200 BC) it is clear that there was a solid and workable body of knowledge relating to energy pathways and the flow of energy through these pathways.

There are many therapeutic arts today, including Shen Tao,

which use as their base this body of knowledge to bring patients into a state of harmony. In many instances healing is directed through pathways or meridians relating to the organs of the body. However, Shen Tao works primarily with the Eight Extraordinary Meridians, which do not relate to specific body organs but to our constitutional or 'core' energy. The Eight Extraordinary Meridians are traditionally likened to lakes and reservoirs (with qualities of depth and stillness) while the organ meridians are likened to rivers (constant flow, movement). Thus Shen Tao, through the Extraordinary Meridians, works directly with the deepest energetic level of being and helps a person to develop a sense of profound inner balance which can then promote the body's natural healing ability.

This natural propensity for self-healing can become blocked, particularly as life in latter-day 20th-century society often creates a high degree of external pressure with little time or space to deal effectively with the resultant stress. So we end up feeling physically unhealthy, emotionally unhappy, mentally confused and spiritually lost.

Shen Tao encourages a return to harmonious living by alleviating the effects of stress as well as by strengthening the core of being. It encourages a deep sense of relaxation and is known to be helpful for difficulties ranging from poor sleep to digestive problems, from muscle or joint pain to depression, anxiety, headaches or blocked creativity.

WHAT TO EXPECT FROM A VISIT TO A THERAPIST

A Shen Tao session starts with a consultation involving Western and Traditional Chinese diagnostic techniques (such as observation of the tongue and pulses) to reach an understanding of the individual and his or her current area of difficulty. This is done by exploring with the patient such things as life patterns, medical history, family patterns, any signs and symptoms of imbalance and so forth. This is followed by a period of 'hands-on' treatment with, wherever possible, time for recovery afterwards. The patient remains clothed throughout. The individual can help before, during and after the session by having a willingness to allow healing or balancing to take place and by being open to exploring any changes which may enhance the healing process. If possible, the patient should avoid eating a heavy meal, taking intoxicants and/or engaging in strenuous activity before and after treatment.

The 'hands-on' treatment aims first to rebalance the general body energies and to strengthen the general constitution, which may have been weakened by, for example, an inappropriate diet, environmental factors, emotional trauma or viral infection at any time in the person's life. Secondly, treatment deals with current or acute symptoms by concentrating on specific areas or points. Finally, treatment is completed by balancing the energy around the shoulders, neck and head. Additional healing techniques may be offered, such as Bach Flower Remedies, visualization, breathing exercises and so forth.

The number of Shen Tao treatments needed will vary according to the needs of the individual concerned.

HOW IT INTERACTS WITH OTHER THERAPIES

Shen Tao combines happily with other complementary and orthodox therapies, although its full benefit may not be appreciated if a patient is receiving a great variety of treatments. If you are already receiving some form of treatment, it may be helpful to consult with the relevant practitioner before embarking upon Shen

Tao. However, you as an individual should ultimately be guided by your own sense of what is appropriate.

QUALIFICATIONS

A Shen Tao Practitioner undertakes a three-year part-time professional training which covers the principles and practice of Traditional Chinese Medicine, Taoist philosophy, anatomy and physiology relevant to the practice of non-invasive Chinese Medicine, with a strong emphasis on the development of intuitive awareness through the study and exploration of subtle energy systems.

By combining the tried-and-tested systems of Traditional Chinese Medicine with a highly developed intuitive awareness, the trained Shen Tao practitioner is able to offer a therapy which respects and honours all beings in a unique way.

NOTE

Shen Tao Acupressure is in its youth and there are currently less than 30 qualified Shen Tao practitioners in Britain and Ireland. In due course, a Shen Tao Register of Practitioners (Dip. Shen Tao) will be constituted. At present, England is the only country which offers a training in Shen Tao.

A list of practitioners and details of their professional training are available from:

The Shen Tao Foundation
c/o Aspects of Health
1 Court Ash
Yeovil
Somerset BA20 1HG
Tel. 0935 410111

Shen Tao forms part of a residential healing programme at:

Middle Piccadilly Natural Healing Centre
Holwell
Nr. Sherborne
Dorset DT9 5LW
Tel. 0963 23468

❧ SHIATSU ❧

HILARY PORTER AND SARA HOOLEY

ORIGINS

Shiatsu, literally meaning 'finger pressure', is both an ancient tradition and a continuing modern development. It evolved out of Chinese massage, one of the four strands of Traditional Chinese Medicine which also includes Acupuncture, moxibustion and herbs. Its still-developing form was officially recognized in Japan earlier this century.

Since time immemorial, touch has been used to show affection, give reassurance and relieve pain. Ancient peoples surely used a form of Shiatsu long before they used the stone and bone implements of early Acupuncture. Originating as a folk remedy (and therefore unrestricted by a formalized academic framework), Shiatsu still maintains the flexibility to respond to the ever-changing needs of people in a developing world.

Currently in the UK, Shiatsu is undergoing a period of intense expansion, reconciling ancient theory with exciting new developments. This accounts for the varying styles of Shiatsu you may experience with different practitioners.

HOW IT WORKS

Shiatsu theory recognizes an energy system in the body. Energy, or *Ki* in Japanese, is most accessible via a network of pathways or meridians which cover the body. Specific points on these meridians (the same as those used in Acupuncture) have a specific action on the Ki. Ki is responsible for the maintenance of all the bodily systems: respiration, digestion, circulation of blood and lymph, the hormones and glands, the central nervous system, the skeleton and the muscles. When the Ki is flowing well, all the body's functions move towards and maintain good health.

Shiatsu is a wonderful combination of energy-balancing and healing touch. Being well-touched from head to foot is a nourishing, relaxing experience for most people. The sense of well-being that results helps to open the meridians, allowing Ki to flow. The body enjoys the physical approach of Shiatsu.

Treatment will includes stretches which also open the meridians. Pressure on the muscles improves the circulation and stimulates the nervous system. By working directly on the meridians, the Shiatsu practitioner can bring the Ki from areas of high energy and redirect it to areas of low energy, restoring balance and the body's ability to heal itself.

What to Expect from a Visit to a Therapist

A Shiatsu session usually lasts an hour, with the practitioner working for 40 to 50 minutes and with time for talk and a rest after treatment. At the first session the practitioner will take a case history, asking a variety of questions covering your reasons for coming, health history and lifestyle. This information, along with that acquired by looking and touching, contributes to the practitioner's understanding of your condition, and so helps him or her to work more effectively.

Treatment usually takes place on a mat on the floor, though it is possible to treat people who are seated in a chair. You will be most comfortable in loose stretchy clothing. Skirts, tight trousers or jeans are not suitable.

Shiatsu involves holding, stretching and applying pressure to the body along the energy pathways, the practitioner using his or her hands, elbows, knees and even feet. The pressure may be strong, but a practitioner may also work very lightly or even away from your body.

After treatment there may be temporary 'healing reactions' as toxins are released, which may take the form of headaches or flu-like symptoms for up to about 24 hours. People generally experience increased well-being and may drift off during treatment into a dreamy state and then, after treatment, feel relaxed and invigorated.

How it Fits into an Individual's Lifestyle

Shiatsu is an Holistic Therapy, and as such addresses each person's problems on a individual level. Some people, who are basically healthy, enjoy the occasional Shiatsu session as a way of relaxing, replenishing their energy and generally maintaining their good health. These people will decide for themselves how often they need or want treatment. If, however, someone has a specific problem which needs addressing, the nature of the problem, its causes and whether it is acute or chronic will all be considered by the practitioner when designing a course of treatments for that individual. For instance, in acute cases a number of weekly or more frequent sessions may be suggested; the patient's progress will be reviewed at each session.

In more chronic cases where someone has been suffering years of discomfort we may recommend that Shiatsu becomes a regular part of that person's life, and that he or she receives treatment once a week, every two weeks or monthly for some time, to bring about a long-term improvement. On the whole, Shiatsu practitioners promote self-responsibility in the people who come to see them. Thus, part of the treatment may be to recommend exercises, dietary changes and even changes in lifestyle, to enable the patient to move towards good health. The practitioner's aim is to help bring about recovery and encourage their patients to develop their own ways of maintaining good health.

WHO CAN BENEFIT?

Shiatsu can be an instant cure if the problem is simple and recent in nature, for example a stiff neck. Very dramatic changes can take place in the course of a single session. Often, though, there is more than one problem to consider. For instance, someone may be suffering from headaches, but then the practitioner's questions may disclose that sleep is also disrupted, the emotions are being tested by relationships at work, constipation has been a long-term problem and that the individual lacks energy. Clearly in such a situation more than one session is called for. The Shiatsu practitioner and patient will constantly review the progress being made, and together work out the treatment programme.

HOW SHIATSU INTERACTS WITH OTHER THERAPIES

Although in itself a complete treatment, some people choose to combine Shiatsu with other therapies. The combination usually works well. Shiatsu is a very good way of getting in touch with emotions and memories that are stored within the body. By opening up the meridians and removing old blocks these emotions can surface and be released. As Shiatsu has a grounding and centring effect, difficult and painful feelings can be acknowledged from a place of safety and security. This capacity to relax, centre and open up makes it very useful in conjunction with Counselling and **Psychotherapy**.

There is a long tradition of using **Herbal Medicine** and Shiatsu together. The pharmacological effects of herbs work on the energy from the inside, while Shiatsu works on the outside. They are mutually supportive and very effective. Shiatsu and **Acupuncture** work within a similar framework and so complement each other well. Each treatment reinforces the other, allowing benefit from both the deep focus of Acupuncture and the touch and movement of Shiatsu as they work together on the energetic structure of the body.

As Shiatsu is a 'touching' therapy it works well with those that are not, but it can also complement the more physical therapies of **Osteopathy** and **Chiropractic**. It is particularly useful before and after a manipulation, helping tense people relax and open up to the treatment, making it more effective. Then, afterwards, Shiatsu helps to maintain the reduction in physical tension brought about by more physical therapies.

Shiatsu can also be very helpful working alongside more conventional forms of treatment. Many people have a series of treatments to support their energy before and after surgery. It also provides a relaxing, energizing and healing treatment for people who are on continuous medication for a chronic or serious disorder.

CONDITIONS FOR WHICH IT IS EFFECTIVE

As Shiatsu affects the energy which underlies all the bodily systems, including the mind and the emotions, it can improve *all* aspects of ill health. It would be impossible to provide a complete list, so here are just a few of the more common ailments relieved by Shiatsu:

- Stress
  Shiatsu's centring and grounding qualities are particularly helpful to people suffering from stress. The practitioner will of course be looking for the cause and help the patient find ways of reducing or eliminating it.
- Headaches
  Headache is a common problem which in the West is most often addressed with pain-killers. Migraine headaches, which can have many different root causes, respond well to Shiatsu.
- Aches, pains, stiffness
  Whether these are caused by arthritis, rheumatism or muscular tension, Shiatsu is very beneficial because of its ability to stimulate the circulation and improve mobility.
- Menstrual problems
  Shiatsu seems to be a very successful way of 'normalizing' the menstrual cycle. This may be partly due to its focus on the Hara (centre, or belly). Other problems associated with the reproductive organs such as impotence, frigidity and premature ejaculation also respond well to treatment.
- General debility
  We often feel lacking in energy and depleted. Shiatsu stimulates the energy flow and is nourishing to the recipient. Patients usually feel energized after a session. Shiatsu helps enormously because of its strengthening qualities.
- Backache
  This is one of the main causes of people having to take time off work in the UK. Shiatsu's holistic approach and hands-on technique make it particularly effective in relieving pain and strengthening the back.
- Injuries
  Broken bones, sprains and bruising all recover more quickly when Shiatsu is used to improve the energy flow through the

injured part. It also addresses the shock associated with such accidents. Once recovery has been gained, the stretches and rotations of Shiatsu help the limbs and joints return to optimum flexibility.

Shiatsu is a wonderful addition to life to help *prevent* ill health; you do not have to be suffering to benefit from it!

QUALIFICATIONS

The Shiatsu Society is an independent regulating body for Shiatsu Practitioners in the UK. It holds a register of practitioners designated by the letters MRSS (Member of the Register of the Shiatsu Society). These practitioners have all reached an approved level of training as established by the Society's assessment panel, and are bound by a code of ethics and a code of practice.

The Shiatsu Society
14 Oakdene Road
Redhill
Surrey RH1 6BT
Tel. 0737 767896

USA
American Oriental Bodywork Therapy Association
50 Maple Place
Manhasset
New York 11030

Further Reading

Chris Jarmey, *Thorsons Introductory Guide to Shiatsu* (Thorsons, 1992)

Chris Jarmey and Gabriel Mojay, *Shiatsu* (Thorsons, 1991)

Wataru Ohashi, *Do-It-Yourself Shiatsu* (Unwin Paperbacks, 1977)

Ray Ridolfi, *Shiatsu* (Optima Alternative Health Series, 1990)

TRADITIONAL
ᔈ CHINESE HERBALISM ᔈ
ALICE LYON

ORIGINS

Chinese Medicine is a complete medical system which has diagnosed, treated and prevented illness for over 23 centuries. There are four basic branches to Chinese Medicine: Herbalism, Food Cures, Acupuncture and Manipulative Therapy. Broadly speaking, Herbalism and Food Cures are part of the system of internal medicine; while Acupuncture and Manipulative Therapy are included in the system of external medicine. The first book on Chinese Healing Arts, the *Nei Ching*, was published in AD 400 and known as the Yellow Emperor's Classics of Internal Medicine; all knowledge of Chinese Medicine stems from this book.

Herbal Medicine uses plants, minerals and animal products prepared in specific ways and combinations to form therapeutic prescriptions. While Chinese Herbs can treat disease states, they also have a large role to play in enhancing immunity, general energy levels and longevity. The medicinal use of Chinese Herbal remedies has well stood the test of time: developed and first used many millennia ago, they are effective for many of today's common disease states. Chinese medicine is based upon clinical experiences over many centuries and such experiences are as valid today as they were centuries ago.

PHILOSOPHY

The strategy of Chinese Medicine is to restore harmony and the goal of treatment to balance Yin and Yang, wet and dry, cold and heat, inner and outer, body and mind. This is achieved by the regulation of *Qi* and of moisture and blood in the organ networks. Qi is the vital energy that travels through us and allows us to move, think and work. Moisture is a liquid that nurtures and lubricates tissue. Blood is the material foundation out of which we create bones, nerves, skin, muscles and organs. The organ networks (liver, heart, spleen, lung and kidney) regulate moisture, blood and Qi, while also governing certain mental faculties and physical activities.

The Chinese system believes that the emotions are connected to these internal organs. Each internal organ is responsible for a specific emotion, and conversely, each emotion acts on a specific internal organ. Thus the heart gives rise to joy, the liver to anger, the lungs to anxiety and sadness, the spleen to worry and thought and the kidneys to fear.

In Western medicine germs and viruses are considered the primary causes of disease. In Chinese medicine the causes of disease are divided into three categories:

1. The Six External Atmospheric Energies: wind, dampness, dryness, heat (fire), cold, and summer heat (a combination of heat and damp or humidity)
2. Internal causes (which include the seven emotions)
3. Fatigue and incorrect foods.

In nature, extreme wind, dampness, dryness, heat and cold can cause chaos in the world. These same forces can upset the balance in the human body, weakening and obstructing it and causing disease.

Wind is in motion and moves constantly, hence when a patient is under the attack of wind the symptoms move around the body, change quickly and seldom last long (an example would be a cold). Wind causes shaking symptoms such as dizziness and muscular twitching.

Dampness is heavy and can cause phlegm or oedema; it is one of the main pathogens causing eczema.

Dryness causes chapping and cracking, constipation, withered and broken hair and dry coughs.

Fire can be seen as inflamed tissue, skin eruptions, ulcers and yellow-green bloody discharges.

The nature of cold is to contract and freeze, so the affected patient will feel cold. Pain is frozen in one place and discharges are clear.

Summer heat is a combination of heat and damp as seen towards the end of the summer; it can manifest as diarrhoea and fevers with profuse sweating.

HOW IT WORKS

Herbal Medicine today uses all the past wealth of information and experience in combination with modern research and knowledge of plants. It is concerned with treating the underlying condition as defined by traditional diagnosis, and rarely causes unwanted side-effects. In fact, the herbs enhance the therapeutic effect of Western drugs so that the dosage of these harsher modern drugs can be lowered and many of their side-effects can be counteracted. This is seen particularly in cancer patients, where the side-effects of Radiotherapy and Chemotherapy are dramatically reduced when Chinese Herbal Medicine forms part of the treatment.

Each herb is categorized in terms of its nature, taste and the particular organ it enters. For example, gold thread, corktree and skullcap are all classified as 'cold' herbs and for that reason are used to treat hot disorders such as infections and inflammatory illnesses, including mastitis, hepatitis and enteritis. On the other hand, cinnamon bark and dried ginger are both 'hot' herbs and are used to treat 'cold' conditions, such as 'cold' arthritis (stiff joints that are cold to the touch and relieved by warmth; the symptoms of 'hot' arthritis would be inflamed, swollen, throbbing joints).

Each flavour we taste affects a different organ. For example, sour flavours are thought to soothe the liver, while sweet flavours work as a tonic for the spleen. Pungent, acrid flavours open up the lungs to clear external pathogens and dry up excess moisture; bitter flavours cool and soothe the heart; salty flavours enter the kidney and soften lumps and nodules.

The taste and therapeutic use of herbs in this way also extends to foods, hence herbal therapy and dietary therapy are prescribed together in Chinese Medicine. If a patient has a hot, inflamed, infected condition, for example, he or she should avoid those foods which would aggravate or worsen symptoms – such as spicy hot foods, fried foods, alcohol and shellfish. For a damp condition like asthma, eczema, sinusitis or obesity, foods that increase the damp pathogens in the body would have to be avoided – for example sweet foods, dairy products and raw foods.

The herbal formulae call for combinations of between two and 14 herbs. The medicine is prescribed in either pill, powder, decoction or extract form. The method of prescribing depends on the condition and the patient's compliance. Individual herbs are treated by frying, charring or soaking in vinegar, salt, etc. in order to enhance their effect or direct them to a particular organ. Charring herbs improves their function of stopping bleeding, for example, while soaking a particular herb in vinegar would allow it to go directly to the liver to work.

WHAT TO EXPECT FROM A VISIT TO A THERAPIST

Herbal Medicine views the body as an organic whole. The outer body and the internal organs are considered to be closely interrelated, hence the traditional diagnostic methods of observing, listening, smelling and palpation. These methods employ, for example, the tongue and pulse as 'maps' to the inner bodily environment. Different areas on the tongue reflect different organs and their condition; when the pulse is palpated it gives information on a person's vital energy and the state of each organ. It is important that each practitioner masters these methods of diagnosis in order to prescribe the correct treatment.

Generally, pills or extracts are prescribed for more chronic conditions while decoctions are given for acute conditions. The duration of treatment will depend on the nature of the problem, its severity and how long it has been affecting the patient. As symptoms improve and the patient makes progress, fewer visits are required. Because Chinese medicine is excellent for both acute and chronic conditions it can be used to replace many commonly prescribed drugs such as antibiotics, aspirin, high blood pressure tablets, etc. It acts more slowly at first than Western drugs, but – especially for chronic conditions – the patient will obtain overall a more lasting and beneficial improvement in health without side-effects and a balance and restoration of inner body harmony.

How it Fits into an Individual's Lifestyle

It is the responsibility of the patient to take the medicine regularly and to follow as closely as possible any dietary advice or other suggestions offered by the practitioner. The herbs work to change the inner environment of the body, both physically and mentally, thereby gently bringing along changes and relief. A prescription used to treat an old person with constipation could also be used to treat a young person with diarrhoea if the cause of both conditions were the same and the same organ weak in a particular way – for example if both were suffering from spleen-deficient Qi.

How it Interacts with Other Therapies

Chinese herbs can be used in conjunction with other closely related therapies such as **Acupuncture** and Chinese Massage. Also, as the herbs allow a gentle mental and emotional change inside the body they can well support any **Psychotherapy** or Counselling treatment.

Conditions for Which it is Effective

As Chinese Medicine until the beginning of the 20th century was the only form of medicine available in China, it was used to treat every disease state. With the introduction of Western medicine many infectious, contagious diseases such as malaria and cholera, and diseases that required surgery began to be treated with Western medicine. As time went on most of the widespread diseases in China were gradually brought under control; however the inadequacies of Western medicine in treating other less threatening but still equally important chronic diseases such as arthritis, heart disease and diabetes were soon realized; Chinese medicine has therefore kept its proper place in health care. In modern China, Chinese and Western medicine are practised side by side and treatment given dependent on patient choice.

Herbs can be used to treat withdrawal symptoms from addictions to sugar, coffee, cigarettes, alcohol, drugs and also for stress reduction, post-surgical recovery, lack of energy and decreased immunity. Infectious illnesses such as colds, flu, bronchitis and hepatitis can be treated with herbs, lessening the need to use antibiotics. Internal organ problems such as hypoglycaemia, asthma, blood pressure, ulcers, colitis, indigestion, haemorrhoids, constipation and diabetes are well controlled by herbal treatment.

Eye, ear, nose and throat problems (such as deafness, ringing in the ears, blurred or poor vision, dizziness, sinus infection, sore throat and hay fever) also respond well to herbal treatment. The use of Chinese Herbs to treat skin diseases such as acne, herpes, etc. has currently been much featured in the media, as these herbs have greatly helped where Western medicine has had very little success.

Musculo-skeletal and neurological problems such as arthritis, neuralgia, back pain, tendonitis, stiff neck, headaches, stroke and sprains are all treated with herbs, which can strengthen the tendons, bones and muscles, clear local inflammation and increase circulation and therefore the nutrition carried to the affected areas. Treatments also help to clear away toxins from the body. External plasters, lotions and herbal pads can also be applied locally to give some pain relief. Herbs greatly help mental and emotional problems, for example anxiety, depression, stress and insomnia, and can be useful to ease patients gently off antidepressants and sleeping tablets so that the side-effects of withdrawal are greatly reduced.

In the reproductive area, traditionally, herbs are used to treat infertility in both men and women, for impotence, pre-menstrual syndrome, irregular periods and cramps, pelvic inflammatory disease, endometriosis, menopause and vaginitis. More recently Herbal Therapy has been seen to counteract the disabling patterns of ME, candida and glandular fever.

The Register of Chinese Herbal Medicine (RCHM)
c/o Alan Treharne
9 Lawns Court
The Avenue
Wembley Park
Middlesex HA9 9PN
Tel. 081–908 1697

Further Reading

Harriet Beinfeld and Efrem Korngold, *Between Heaven and Earth: A Guide to Chinese Medicine* (Ballantine, 1991)

Dr Stephen T. Chang, *The Complete System of Chinese Self-healing* (Aquarian, 1994)

Ted Kaptchuk, *The Web That Has No Weaver* (New York: Condon & Weed, 1983)

❧ WESTERN HERBAL MEDICINE ❧

SUE EVANS

ORIGINS

The use of therapeutic herbs goes back beyond written records. Early man, from his own experience and from watching the instinctive habits of animals, would have come to realize that certain plants were beneficial for the ailments that plagued him while others seemed to be of no value at all, or even potentially fatal! There must have been a good deal of trial and error in these early experiments.

Our first records of herbal use date from around 2500 BC, but these Sumerian and Assyrian records are unfortunately incomplete. It is the Greek and Roman civilizations to whom we owe more detailed information of the progress of Western Herbalism. The Greek doctor Hippocrates listed over 400 herbs in use in the healing temples, or *Aesculapions*, of that era, many of which are still in use today. The philosopher Aristotle also studied the use of herbs and compiled one of the first recorded classifications of herbs according to their action in the body.

When the Romans invaded Britain they brought many of their own native herbs with them for use when the legions fell sick; these herbs and the knowledge of their use were incorporated into the herbal lore of the native Britons. Other herbs were introduced in a similar fashion, the next major influx being during the sea explorations of Elizabethan England when many herbs from the American continent were introduced. These were the days when all big houses had their own herb gardens, many of which still survive today, for treating the ills of the household. The Chelsea

Physic Garden was developed by the Society of Apothecaries in 1673 inspired by Henry Lyte, whose earlier garden had attracted much attention.

The major difference between Chinese or Oriental Herbalism and Western Herbalism is the way in which the herbs are classified as to their action in the body. The concepts of Oriental herbal medicine are more energetic in nature: herbs are classified according to their properties of heating, cooling, moistening, drying, of moving energy into the system or driving it out, depending on the perceived imbalance in the patient. Many of the same herbs are used in Western Herbalism, but the ways in which they are prepared may differ.

PHILOSOPHY

In the early days of Western Herbal lore we find reference to a classification of herbs similar to that of Oriental Herbalism. Nicholas Culpepper (1616–54) wrote of energetic principles, of heating and cooling herbs. He also associated herbs with certain planets, claiming for those herbs governed by a particular planet the properties attributed astrologically to the planet itself. Most of this energetic knowledge has been lost to us in the West and is just being revived by the work and studies of modern herbalists, although much of it remains implicit in the traditional combinations of herbs for certain conditions.

HOW IT WORKS

Today Western Herbalism classifies herbs according to their action in the body in a similar manner to the way in which they were recorded by Aristotle in the 4th century BC. There are herbs which are, for instance:

- astringent, condensing tissues which have become too lax
- anti-spasmodics, which prevent the recurrence of spasms
- demulcents, which soothe and cool inflamed or injured tissue
- tonics, which strengthen the whole system (often by working on the endocrine glands)
- alteratives, which cleanse the bloodstream
- relaxants, hepatics, stimulants and many more.

Their actions are not merely imposed upon the body in an aggressive or suppressive fashion, they are chosen to work with the body to bring about a state of harmony and balance within the system, which is then maintained. Much of the action is nutritive, the herb supplying the tissues with the nutrients they need to heal, build, repair and restore normal function, although certain substances in the plants also augment and support this nutritive action.

Many of the causes of imbalance in the body relate to congestion of the system, the build-up of toxins in the body due to inadequate nutrition, underfunction of the organs of elimination, etc. Before the system can be strengthened and balanced, these toxins must be removed. There is often, therefore, a need for a period of cleansing using herbs to stimulate the detoxifying action of the liver, the colon, the lymph, the lungs and skin. During detoxification weaker organs may have to be supported, for example, the heart and one's susceptibility to stress may need to be reduced; in this case the formula may include nervine herbs and circulatory tonics. A focus of infection may need to be dealt with and here the use of alterative, anti-microbial and immune-enhancing herbs would be recommended.

Creating a herbal formula for a patient requires a compound knowledge of the causes of the underlying problem and also of the specific properties of the herbs employed. Since we are not composed only of our physical bodies but are also very much affected by emotional states, truly holistic treatment must take this into account. It is true that in releasing toxins from the body and rebalancing particularly the glandular system, much negative emotion is also released. This allows the emotions to become more stable generally. Many herbalists will use Bach Flower Remedies as a natural complement to herbal treatment.

WHAT TO EXPECT FROM A VISIT TO A HERBALIST

During a herbal consultation a full case history is taken: family history, record of past illnesses, present complaint, etc. There will also be questions about the nature of your work, leisure time activities, eating habits, etc. to eliminate circumstantial or environmental factors contributing to your particular health problem. The Herbalist will also need to get to know you as a person, where the underlying emotional tensions are, how you relate to life, your experiences, what affects you profoundly – this again helps to form a complete picture of you as a patient and allows for a truly holistic treatment.

Usually during the consultation there will be a physical examination: blood pressure, resting pulse rate, palpation of the abdomen, etc. depending on the particular case. Sometimes the physical examination may be augmented or replaced by other methods of analysis, such as pulse diagnosis, iridology, etc. according to the training of the Herbalist.

CONDITIONS FOR WHICH IT IS EFFECTIVE

Herbal Medicine can be used to treat a great variety of problems – it was, after all, the mainstream medicine of its time and many of our elder generation can still remember being given medicines based on herbs. Having said this, it is particularly effective for gastro-intestinal problems, problems relating to stress and menstrual and endocrine problems, to name but a few.

Herbs offer a powerful source of healing for the body when used in the right way. They should never be treated casually as a harmless and mildly eccentric form of treatment. Some of the medical professions' most potent drugs have been extracted from herbs and plants, which remain one of the primary potential sources of new medicines. Herbalists believe that the therapeutic properties of a plant are best left in combination, as nature intended, with other synergistic and modifying substances to provide a well-balanced treatment for the human body. Even then, some herbs can have unpleasant or dangerous side-effects if the recommended dosage is exceeded or if they are used inappropriately. Too strong a cleansing action on a weak or over-toxic body system can have uncomfortable effects at best.

However, many plants can be safely and frequently used on a daily basis for relaxation; Chamomile and lime flower teas are effective for minor ills; an elderflower and peppermint infusion combats mild flu; dandelion and burdock act as a cleanser for the body. As you can see, these combinations are common knowledge to most and were frequently employed not so many years ago. Used properly, herbs will gently bring the body into a better state of balance and harmony, treating even long-term and chronic conditions at a pace consistent with the natural laws of healing. They can then be used, once this balance has been attained, to maintain the equilibrium of the system through the various pressures life imposes, thus ensuring better health for this and succeeding generations.

How it Fits into an Individual's Lifestyle

Herbalism is a therapy which calls for the commitment of the patient to a course of treatment; little will be gained by a half-hearted attitude. If the herbs are not taken as directed or if additional advice regarding diet, etc. is not followed, results may be poor. Sometimes the benefits can be seen very early on, such as is often the case with menstrual discomfort and certain types of headache; other problems which have built up over a number of months and years, however, will take a correspondingly longer time to clear. Perseverance to a course of treatment will bring the desired effect at the body's natural pace.

Because of the principles of Herbalism, which are based on cleansing and then rebalancing the system, there may be a period of aggravation in some cases as toxins are released from the system. Generally the practitioner will try to make treatment as trouble-free as possible, but even if 'crises' occur they should be welcomed in the knowledge that the toxins are moving out of the system and the episode will leave the patient experiencing a new level of health.

Qualifications

The main Herbal training college in the UK is the National Institute of Medical Herbalists. Graduates have the initials MNIMH and have studied for a minimum of four years. Dr Christopher's American School of Herbology confers the initials MH on graduates who have also undergone extensive training in the principles of Naturopathic and herbal healing. Graduates of the British School of Iridology (MBRI) are also trained in the use of herbs and Naturopathy according to the principles laid down by Dr

Christopher. Other Colleges such as Michael Tierra's Herbal College give an excellent training, using knowledge from Chinese, ayurvedic, Native American and European herbal schools. Kitty Campion's Herbal College in Newcastle-under-Lyme also offers training in herbal and Naturopathic therapies.

The General Council and Register of Consultant Herbalists
Grosvenor House
40 Seaway
Middleton-on-Sea
Sussex PO22 7SA
Tel. 0243 586012

National Institute of Medical Herbalists
9 Palace Gate
Exeter
Devon EX1 1JA
Tel. 0392 426022

Australia
Australian Traditional Medicine Society
120 Blaxland Road
Ryde NSW 2112
Tel. 808 2825

National Herbalists Association of Australia
14/249 Kingsgrove Road
Kingsgrove NSW 2208
Tel. 502 2938

USA
California School of Herbal Studies
PO Box 39
Forestville, CA 95436
Tel. 707–887–7457

Flower Essence Society
PO Box 1769
Nevada City, CA 95959
Tel. 916–265–9163

Further Reading

John R. Christopher, *School of Natural Healing* (Provo, UT: Biworld Publishers, 1979)

Nalda Gosling, *Successful Herbal Remedies* (Thorsons, 1993)

David Hoffmann, *The New Holistic Herbal* (Element Books, 1990)

—, *Thorsons Guide to Medical Herbalism* (Thorsons, 1991)

Simon Mills, *The Complete Guide to Modern Herbalism* (Thorsons, 1994)

Michael Tierra, *Planetary Herbology* (Twin Lakes, WI: Lotus, 1988)

—, *The Way of Herbs* (Pocket Books, 1990)

PART FOUR

WHICH THERAPY?

Introduction to
❧ the Reference Charts ❧

These reference charts can help to guide readers to the therapy or therapies that they should consider when contemplating treatment for a particular complaint.

Many therapies indicated for a particular condition are often best used in tandem with other therapies. For best results it may be necessary to use a mixture of two or more therapies to gain the best results. This is especially true for conditions that are exacerbated by stress. On the other hand, some therapies are *not* compatible, such as Homoeopathy and Aromatherapy: the volatile oils used in Aromatherapy can negate the effects of homoeopathic remedies. Always check with a therapist or practitioner whether his or her therapy can be used in combination with another/others.

Many techniques suggested (e.g. massage for children suffering from sleep problems) can be learned on short courses or from self-help books and practised by parents at home.

Any lumps should always be investigated fully, the necessary tests being taken to determine the nature of the lump before seeking treatment.

The 12 charts are broken down into these problem areas:

Accidents and injuries
Children's problems
Cardiovascular system
Respiratory system
Nervous system/emotional disorders
Endocrine system

Reproductive system (women's problems, then men's)
Digestive system
Urinary system
Skin problems
Musculo-skeletal system
Special senses (ears, nose, eyes, mouth)

The left–hand (vertical) column of each chart specifies particular complaints, such as bites/stings in the chart dealing generally with accidents and injuries. The right–hand (horizontal) column lists the therapies discussed in this book which can help to treat the complaint (in the case of bites/stings, for example, Acupuncture, Aromatherapy, Herbalism and Homoeopathy are all options you might consider).

Please note:

- Acupressure includes the Shen Tao form of this therapy.
  The term Aromatherapy in the context of these charts includes the practice of using essential oils in a variety of ways – in massage, added to the bath, etc.
- Counselling refers to Psychotherapy as well as other forms of personal counselling.
- Herbalism can be taken to include Chinese as well as Western forms of this therapy.
- Iridology is frequently considered to be a diagnostic aid rather than a specific treatment. It can help to determine which body systems are weak or in need of support from other types of therapy, the source (within the body) of a complaint, and which areas should be further investigated. For example, tinnitus may be due to an inner ear problem or to cervical vertebra misalignment. Iridology may well be able to pinpoint causes while not necessarily being able to treat specific problems.
- Massage includes the therapies Relaxation Massage, Remedial Massage and Rosen Method Bodywork.

- The term Osteopathy in the context of these charts incorporates Cranial Osteopathy.

If in doubt about choosing a therapy to match a particular complaint, expert guidance should be sought.

Disorders to Different Body Systems, and Therapy Options

Wounds	Travel sickness	Sunburn	Sprains/Strains	Shock	Nosebleeds	Fainting	Eye injuries	Burns/Scald	Bruises	Blisters	Bites/Stings	ACCIDENTS AND INJURIES
			×						×			Acupressure
	×		×	×	×	×	×		×		×	Acupuncture
			×	×								Applied Kinesiology
×	×	×	×	×					×	×	×	Aromatherapy Essential Oils
				×		×						Bach Flower Remedies
			×									Chiropractic
				×								Counselling
			×	×			×					Healing
×	×	×	×	×	×	×	×	×	×	×	×	Herbalism
×	×	×	×	×	×	×	×	×	×	×	×	Homoeopathy
	×											Hypnotherapy
			×	×					×			Massage
	×											Neuro-Linguistic Programming
	×											Naturopathy
	×											Nutrition and Diet
			×									Osteopathy
				×								Polarity
				×								Psychotherapy
			×		×							Reflexology
			×						×			Shiatsu

Therapy	Teething/toothache	Sore throats	Sleep problems	Nappy Rash	Mumps	Measles	Hyperactivity	Glue ear	German Measles	Fever	Eye inflammations	Eczema	Earache	Coughs	Constipation	Colic	Colds & Catarrh	Chicken pox	Chest infections	Behaviour problems	Bedwetting	Anxiety	Adenoids
Acupressure			×																			×	
Acupuncture	×		×	×	×	×	×	×	×	×	×	×	×	×	×	×	×	×	×	×	×	×	×
Applied Kinesiology		×	×				×	×				×		×	×	×	×		×	×		×	×
Aromatherapy Essential Oils	×	×	×	×	×	×	×			×	×		×	×	×	×	×	×	×	×		×	
Bach Flower Remedies			×				×													×		×	
Chiropractic															×						×		
Colour therapy			×				×													×		×	
Counselling			×																	×	×	×	
Healing			×				×	×		×		×	×	×	×	×	×		×	×	×	×	
Herbalism	×	×	×	×	×	×	×	×	×	×	×	×	×	×	×	×	×	×	×	×	×	×	×
Homoeopathy	×	×	×	×	×	×	×	×	×	×	×	×	×	×	×	×	×	×	×	×	×	×	×
Hypnotherapy			×																	×	×		
Iridology		×	×				×					×	×	×	×	×			×	×	×		
Massage			×																			×	
Naturopathy			×				×	×				×	×		×	×	×		×	×		×	×
Nutrition and Diet			×				×	×				×	×		×	×	×		×	×		×	×
Osteopathy			×					×					×		×	×	×		×	×			
Psychotherapy			×																	×	×	×	
Reflexology	×		×				×	×						×	×	×	×		×			×	×
Shiatsu			×																			×	

Varicose Veins	Varicose Ulcers	Circulation (Poor)	Blood pressure (Hyper or Hypotension)	Arteriosclerosis (Hardening of the arteries)	Anaemia	CARDIO-VASCULAR SYSTEM
×		×	×			Acupressure
×		×	×			Acupuncture
×		×	×		×	Applied Kinesiology
×		×	×			Aromatherapy Essential Oils
			×			Autogenic Training
	×		×			Healing
×	×	×	×	×	×	Herbalism
×	×	×	×	×	×	Homoeopathy
			×			Hypnotherapy
		×			×	Iridology
×		×	×			Massage
		×	×		×	Naturopathy
			×			Neuro-Linguistic Programming
		×	×		×	Nutrition and Diet
×		×	×			Osteopathy
		×	×			Polarity
		×	×			Reflexology
		×	×			Shiatsu

Tracheitis	Sore throats	Sinusitis	Pleurisy	Hay fever	Coughs	Colds	Bronchitis	Asthma	RESPIRATORY SYSTEM
		x					x	x	Acupressure
x	x	x	x	x	x	x	x	x	Acupuncture
								x	Alexander Technique
	x	x			x	x	x	x	Applied Kinesiology
x	x	x	x	x		x	x	x	Aromatherapy
								x	Autogenic Training
								x	Bach Flower Remedies
								x	Chiropractic
								x	Colour therapy
								x	Counselling
		x	x		x		x	x	Healing
x	x	x	x	x	x	x	x	x	Herbalism
x	x	x	x	x	x	x	x	x	Homoeopathy
								x	Hypnotherapy
								x	Massage
		x		x		x	x	x	Naturopathy
								x	Neuro-Linguistic Programming
		x		x		x	x	x	Nutrition and Diet
								x	Osteopathy
								x	Polarity
								x	Psychotherapy
x	x	x	x			x	x	x	Reflexology
								x	Rolfing
							x	x	Shiatsu

NERVOUS SYSTEM/ EMOTIONAL DISORDERS

	Trauma	Trapped Nerves	Shingles	Sciatica	Neuralgia	M.E.	Headaches	Fainting	Epilepsy	Dizziness	Carpal Tunnel Syndrome	Bell's Palsy	Alzheimer's	Trauma	Stress	Schizophrenia	Phobias	Insomnia	Grief	Depression	Anxiety	Anorexia/Bulimia	Addictions
Acupressure	×			×			×								×			×		×	×		
Acupuncture	×	×	×	×	×	×	×	×	×	×	×		×	×	×	×	×	×	×	×	×	×	×
Alexander Technique	×						×								×						×		
Applied Kinesiology	×	×		×	×	×	×			×			×	×	×	×	×	×	×	×	×	×	×
Aromatherapy	×		×	×	×	×	×						×		×			×	×	×	×		
Autogenic Training	×						×							×	×		×	×	×	×	×	×	×
Bach Flower Remedies	×						×	×	×	×				×	×		×	×	×	×	×	×	×
Chiropractic	×	×		×	×		×	×	×	×	×	×		×	×								
Colour therapy	×													×	×		×	×	×	×			
Counselling	×						×							×	×	×	×	×	×	×	×	×	×
Healing	×	×	×	×	×	×	×	×	×	×	×		×	×	×	×	×	×	×	×	×		
Herbalism			×		×	×	×	×	×	×		×	×	×	×		×	×	×	×	×	×	×
Homoeopathy	×		×		×	×	×	×	×	×	×		×	×	×	×	×	×	×	×	×	×	×
Hypnotherapy	×						×							×	×	×	×	×	×	×	×	×	×
Iridology						×	×	×		×													
Massage	×			×			×								×			×			×		
Naturopathy						×	×	×		×												×	
Neuro-Linguistic Programming	×													×	×		×	×	×	×	×	×	×
Nutrition and Diet						×	×	×		×										×		×	
Osteopathy	×	×		×	×		×	×	×	×	×	×		×	×								
Polarity	×				×	×	×							×	×			×		×	×	×	
Psychotherapy	×						×							×	×	×	×	×	×	×	×	×	×
Reflexology	×				×	×	×			×					×			×					
Rolfing	×			×			×								×			×					
Shiatsu	×			×			×								×			×			×		

Weight Loss/Gain	Recurrent Infections	Obesity	Hypoglycaemia	Hyperlipidaemia (High Cholesterol)	Hyper or Hypo Thyroidism	Fatigue/Lassitude	Diabetes	ENDOCRINE SYSTEM GENERAL
						×		Acupressure
×	×	×	×	×	×	×	×	Acupuncture
×	×	×	×	×	×	×	×	Applied Kinesiology
	×				×	×		Aromatherapy
×		×						Autogenic Training
×		×						Bach Flower Remedies
×		×				×		Colour therapy
×		×						Counselling
	×					×	×	Healing
×	×	×	×	×	×	×	×	Herbalism
×	×		×	×	×	×	×	Homoeopathy
×		×						Hypnotherapy
	×		×	×	×	×	×	Iridology
						×		Massage
×	×	×	×	×		×	×	Naturopathy
×		×						Neuro-Linguistic Programming
×	×	×	×	×		×	×	Nutrition and Diet
						×		Osteopathy
×		×	×	×		×	×	Polarity
×		×						Psychotherapy
	×				×	×	×	Reflexology
						×		Rolfing
						×		Shiatsu

REPRODUCTIVE SYSTEM

Therapy	Sexual Problems (M)	Sexually Transmitted Diseases (M)	Prostate	Inflammation of Testes	Impotence	Genital Herpes (M)	Useful in Pregnancy	Vaginitis	Sexually Transmitted Diseases (F)	Menstrual Problems	Menopause	Infertility	Genital Herpes (F)	Fibroids	Endometriosis	Candida	Mastitis	Lumps	Cysts	Breasts: Abcess	Sexual Problems (F)
Acupressure										×		×				×					
Acupuncture		×	×	×	×	×	×	×	×	×	×	×	×	×	×	×	×	×	×	×	×
Applied Kinesiology	×		×			×				×	×	×			×	×		×			
Aromatherapy			×	×	×	×	×	×		×	×	×	×		×	×	×	×	×	×	
Autogenic Training	×																				×
Bach Flower Remedies	×				×		×			×	×	×									×
Colour therapy					×		×			×	×	×									
Counselling	×	×			×		×		×	×	×										×
Healing			×	×	×					×	×	×			×	×		×	×	×	
Herbalism		×	×	×	×	×	×	×	×	×	×	×	×	×	×	×	×	×	×		
Homoeopathy	×	×	×	×	×	×	×	×	×	×	×	×	×	×	×	×	×	×	×	×	×
Hypnotherapy	×				×						×	×									×
Iridology					×		×			×		×				×					
Massage							×			×						×					
Naturopathy							×			×	×				×						
Neuro-Linguistic Programming	×				×						×										×
Nutrition and Diet							×			×	×				×						
Polarity	×				×		×			×	×	×		×		×					×
Psychotherapy	×				×						×	×									×
Reflexology							×			×	×	×		×	×	×			×		
Shiatsu							×			×						×					

Worms	Vomiting	Ulcers	Oesophagitis	Nausea	Irritable Bowel	Indigestion	Hepatitis	Haemorrhoids	Gastroenteritis	Gastritis, Acute or Chronic	Gallstones	Diverticulitis	Distension	Constipation	Colic	Appetite - Bulimia/Anorexia	DIGESTIVE SYSTEM
						×							×	×	×	×	Acupressure
	×	×	×	×	×	×	×	×	×	×	×	×	×	×	×	×	Acupuncture
	×	×		×	×	×				×	×	×	×	×	×	×	Applied Kinesiology
			×	×	×	×	×	×	×	×	×		×	×	×	×	Aromatherapy Essential Oils
																×	Autogenic Training
				×												×	Bach Flower Remedies
								×						×			Chiropractic
												×	×	×	×	×	Colour therapy
		×		×												×	Counselling
		×	×	×	×	×	×			×	×	×	×	×			Healing
×	×	×	×	×	×	×	×	×	×	×	×	×	×	×	×	×	Herbalism
×	×	×	×	×	×	×	×	×	×	×	×	×	×	×	×	×	Homoeopathy
																×	Hypnotherapy
					×	×							×				Iridology
	×	×	×	×	×	×	×	×	×	×	×	×	×	×	×	×	Naturopathy
					×											×	Neuro-Linguistic Programming
	×	×	×	×	×	×		×	×	×	×	×	×		×	×	Nutrition and Diet
								×						×			Osteopathy
		×	×		×	×	×	×		×	×	×	×	×	×	×	Polarity
					×											×	Psychotherapy
	×	×	×	×	×	×	×	×	×	×	×	×	×	×	×	×	Reflexology
					×	×							×	×			Rolfing
					×								×	×	×		Shiatsu

URINARY SYSTEM

Water Retention	Chronic	Renal Failure	Painful Urination	Kidney Stones	Irritable Bladder	Frequency of Urination	Cystitis	Bedwetting	
×									Acupressure
×	×	×		×	×	×	×	×	Acupuncture
×	×	×	×	×	×	×	×	×	Applied Kinesiology
×			×	×	×	×	×	×	Aromatherapy Essential Oils
								×	Autogenic Training
								×	Bach Flower Remedies
					×	×		×	Chiropractic
					×			×	Colour therapy
								×	Counselling
×	×	×	×	×	×	×	×	×	Healing
×	×	×	×	×	×	×	×	×	Herbalism
×	×	×	×	×	×	×	×	×	Homoeopathy
								×	Hypnotherapy
×					×			×	Iridology
×	×		×				×		Naturopathy
								×	Neuro-Linguistic Programming
×	×		×				×		Nutrition and Diet
×					×	×		×	Osteopathy
×	×		×				×		Polarity
								×	Psychotherapy
×	×	×		×	×	×	×	×	Reflexology
×									Shiatsu

Warts	Urticaria	Ulcers	Ring Worm	Psoriasis	Greasy Skin	Exessive Perspiration	Eczema	Cysts	Cracks/Fissures	Cold Sores	Chilblains	Cellulite	Boils/Carbuncles	Athletes Foot	Alopecia	Acne	Abcesses	SKIN PROBLEMS
		x									x	x						Acupressure
			x	x	x	x	x			x	x				x	x	x	Acupuncture
	x	x		x		x	x									x		Applied Kinesiology
x	x	x	x	x	x	x	x	x	x	x	x	x	x	x	x	x	x	Aromatherapy
																x		Colour therapy
				x			x									x		Counselling
x		x		x			x	x								x	x	Healing
x	x	x	x	x	x	x	x	x	x	x	x	x	x	x	x	x	x	Herbalism
x	x	x	x	x	x	x	x	x	x	x	x	x	x	x	x	x	x	Homoeopathy
																x		Hypnotherapy
					x	x				x	x	x	x			x	x	Iridology
		x									x	x				x		Massage
x	x	x	x	x	x	x	x			x	x	x	x	x	x	x	x	Naturopathy
x	x	x	x	x	x	x	x			x	x	x	x	x	x	x	x	Nutrition and Diet
x	x	x	x	x	x	x	x			x	x	x	x	x	x		x	Polarity
																x		Psychotherapy
		x		x	x	x	x			x	x	x				x	x	Reflexology
	x										x	x						Shiatsu

MUSCULO-SKELETAL SYSTEM

	Trapped nerve	Tenosynovitis	Sciatica	Rheumatism	Pagets Disease	Osteoporosis	Neck Problems	Muscles, Pulled or Strained	Lumbago	Arm	Hip/Knee	Ankle/Elbow	Joint Problems,	Hernias	Gout	General Back Problems	Ganglions	Fibrositis	Disc Problems	Cramp	Cervical Spondylosis	Bursitis	Arthritis, Osteo or Rheumatoid	Ankylosing Spondylitis
Acupressure	×	×	×	×			×	×	×	×	×		×			×			×	×			×	
Acupuncture	×	×	×	×	×	×	×	×	×	×	×		×		×	×		×	×	×	×	×	×	×
Alexander Technique	×		×				×									×			×					
Applied Kinesiology						×	×	×	×	×	×		×	×		×				×	×		×	
Aromatherapy			×	×			×	×	×							×		×		×			×	
Chiropractic	×	×	×	×			×	×	×	×	×		×			×		×	×	×	×	×	×	×
Healing	×	×	×	×			×	×	×	×	×		×			×		×		×			×	
Herbalism				×		×		×	×	×	×		×		×	×		×	×	×	×		×	
Homoeopathy				×		×		×	×	×	×		×		×	×		×	×	×	×		×	
Massage			×	×			×	×	×	×	×		×			×		×	×	×			×	
Naturopathy															×	×					×		×	
Nutrition and Diet															×	×					×		×	
Osteopathy	×	×	×	×	×	×	×	×	×	×	×		×			×		×	×	×	×	×	×	×
Polarity							×								×	×					×		×	
Reflexology									×												×			
Rolfing	×	×	×	×			×	×	×	×	×		×			×		×	×	×				
Shiatsu	×	×	×	×				×	×	×	×		×			×		×	×	×			×	

SPECIAL SENSES

Condition	Acupuncture	Applied Kinesiology	Aromatherapy	Chiropractic	Healing	Herbalism	Homoeopathy	Naturopathy	Nutrition and Diet	Osteopathy	Polarity	Reflexology	Rolfing
EYE:													
Astigmatism													
Blepharitis						×	×						
Cataracts						×	×						
Conjunctivitis						×	×						
Eye Strain					×								
Foreign Bodies					×	×	×						
Injury/Trauma						×	×						
Sight, Short, Long, Squint													
Styes, Cysts						×	×						
Twitching Eyelids	×					×	×						
Watering Eyes	×					×	×						
MOUTH													
Burning Mouth Syndrome	×					×	×	×	×				
Candida (Thrush)		×				×	×						
Gingivitis		×				×	×						
Gum Boils/Abcesses	×					×	×	×	×				
Halitosis	×					×	×						
Herpes Simplex						×	×						
Stomatitis						×	×						
Teething/Toothache	×					×	×						
Ulcers	×					×	×						

Sinusitis	Rhinitis	Hay Fever	Epistaxis (Nose Bleeds)	Catarrh	NOSE	Wax	Vertigo	Tinnitus	Otitis Media	Menierés Disease	Mastoiditis	Labyrinthitis	Ear, Tube Blockage	Eustachian, Glue	Earache	EAR: SPECIAL SENSES
×	×	×	×	×		×	×	×	×	×		×		×	×	Acupuncture
×	×	×		×		×										Applied Kinesiology
×	×			×			×								×	Aromatherapy
×	×						×	×		×				×		Chiropractic
							×	×		×				×		Healing
×	×	×	×	×				×	×	×	×	×		×		Herbalism
×	×	×	×	×		×	×	×	×	×	×	×	×	×	×	Homoeopathy
×	×			×										×		Naturopathy
×	×			×										×		Nutrition and Diet
×	×						×	×		×				×		Osteopathy
				×			×									Polarity
				×												Reflexology
							×									Rolfing

INDEX OF
PROFESSIONAL QUALIFICATIONS

AHPP	Association of Humanistic Psychology Practitioners
AIPTI	Association of Independent Professional Therapists International
AIRMT	Associate of the International Register of Manipulative Therapists
AMA	Anthroposophical Medical Association
AMP	Association of Massage Practitioners
ANLP	Association for Neuro-Linguistic Programming
ATA	Associate of Tisserand Aromatherapists
BAAR	British Acupuncture Association & Register
BAc	Bachelor of Acupuncture
BAC	British Association of Counsellors
BAHA	British Alliance of Healing Associations
BALCCH	London College of Classical Homoeopathy
BAThH	British Association of Therapeutic Hypnosis
BCA	British Chiropractic Association
BCHE	British Council of Hypnotherapy Examiners
BH (Hons)	Bachelor of Humanities (University of London)
BHMA	British Holistic Medicine Association
Biod.Phys	Biodynamic Psychiatrist
BMAS	British Medical Acupuncture Society (doctors only)
BPS	British Psychological Society
BRS	British Rebirth Society
BS	Bachelor of Surgery
BSD	British Society of Dowsers

BWOY	British Wheel of Yoga
CAc	Certificate of Acupuncture (China)
CCAc	Certificate in Chinese Acupressure
CCAM	Council for Complementary and Alternative Medicine
Cert HS	Certificate in Herbal Studies
CfA	Council for Acupuncture
CHP	Certificate in Hypnotherapy & Psychotherapy (from the National College of Hypnosis & Psychotherapy)
CHyp	Council of Hypnotherapists
CQSW	Certificate of Qualification in Social Work
CSAS	Chung San Acupuncture Society
DAc	Diploma in Acupuncture (College of Traditional Chinese Acupuncture)
DC	Diploma in Chiropractic
DCH	Diploma of Child Health
DHM	Diploma in Holistic Medicine
D.Hom	Diploma in Homoeopathy
DHP	Diploma in Hypnotherapy & Psychotherapy
Dip BWT	British Wheel of Yoga Diploma
Dip C	Diploma in Counselling
Dip Hyp	Diploma of Hypnotherapy
Dip PC	Diploma in Psychic Counselling
Dip Phyt	Diploma in Phytotherapy (herbal medicine)
Dip THP	Diploma in Therapeutic Hypnosis & Psychotherapy
DN	Diploma in Nursing
DO	Diploma in Osteopathy
DobstRCOG	Diploma from Royal College of Obstetricians & Gynaecologists
DPH	Diploma in Public Health
DPM	Diploma in Psychological Medicine

DrAc	Doctor of Acupuncture (from the British College of Acupuncture)
DSH	Diploma from the School of Homoeopathy
DThD	Diploma in Dietary Therapy
DTM	Diploma in Therapeutic Massage awarded by London College of Holistic Medicine
FBAcA	Fellow of the British Acupuncture Association
FBRA	Fellow of the British Reflexology Association
FCOS	Fellow of the College of Ophthalmic Somatology
FFHom	Fellow of the Faculty of Homoeopathy
FHSMS	Fellow of the Henderson School of Manipulative Surgery
FIH	Fellow of the Indian Institute of Homoeopathy
FIHP	Fellow of the Institute of Hypnosis & Parapsychology
FIMLS	Fellow of the Institute of Medical Laboratory Science
FRCSG	Fellow of the Royal College of Physicians, Glasgow
FRH	Fellow of the Register of Herbalists (from the General Council & Register of Hypnosis & Psychotherapy)
IROM	International Register of Oriental Medicine
ISPA	International Society of Practising Aromatherapists
ITEC	International Therapy Examination Council
LCCH	London College of Classical Homoeopathy
LCH	Licentiate of the College of Homoeopathy
LCSP	London & Counties Society of Physiologists
LCSP(Assoc)	Associate of London & Counties Society of Physiology
LCSP(BTh)	London & Counties Society of Physiologists (Beauty Therapeutics)
LCSP(DO)	London & Counties Society of Physiologists (Osteopathy)

LCSP.Phys	London & Counties Society of Physiologists (Manipulative Therapy)
LDS	Licentiate in Dental Surgery
LGSM	Licentiate of the Guildhall School of Music
LicAc	Licentiate of Acupuncture
LLSA	Licentiate of the London School of Aromatherapy
LNCP	Licentiate Member of the National Council of Psychotherapists & Hypnotherapy Register
LRCP	Licentiate of the Royal College of Physicians
MAA	Member of the Auricular Therapy Association
MABP	Member of the Association of Biodynamic Psychotherapists
MAc	Master of Acupuncture (diploma awarded by the College of Traditional Chinese Acupuncture and by the International College of Oriental Medicine [ICOM])
MACH	Member of the Association of Classical Hypnotherapists
MAHPP	Member of the Association of Humanistic Psychology Practitioners
MAPT	Member of the Association of Professional Therapists
MAQCH	Member of the Association of Qualified Curative Hypnotherapists
MAR	Member of the Association of Reflexologists
MAWAc	Member of the Association of Western Acupuncture
MB	Bachelor of Medicine
MBAcA	Member of the British Acupuncture Association
MBBS	Bachelor of Medicine & Surgery
MBEOA	Member of the British and European Osteopathic Association
MBNOA	Member of the British Naturopathic & Osteopathic Association

MBRA	Member of the British Reflexology Association
MBSAM	Member of the British School of Acupressure
MBSH	Member of the British Society of Hypnotherapists
MBSR	Member of the British School of Reflexology
MC	McTimony Chiropractor
MCH	Member of the College of Homoeopathy
MCO	Member of the College of Osteopaths
MCOA	Member of the Cranial Osteopath Association
MCOS	Member of the College of Ophthalmic Somatology
MCROA	Member of the Cranial Osteopathic Association
MCSAcS	Member of Chung San Acupuncture Society
MCSP	Member of the Chartered Society of Physiotherapists
MFG	Member of the Feldenkrais Guild
MFHom	Member of the Faculty of Homoeopathy
MFPhys	Member of the Faculty of Physiatrists
MGO	Member of the Guild of Osteopathy
MH	Master Herbalist
MHMA(UK)	Member of the United Kingdom Medical Association
MHPA	Member of the Health Practitioners Association
MIAC	Member of the Institute of Applied Osteopathy
MIACT	Member of the International Association of Colour Therapists
MIAH	Member of the Institute of Analytical Hypnotherapists
MICH	Member of the Institute of Curative Hypnotherapists
MIFA	Member of the International Federation of Aromatherapists
MIGN(med)	Member of the International Guild of Natural Medicine Practitioners

MIIR	Member of the International Institute of Reflexology
MInstAT	Member of the Institute of Allergy Therapists
MIPC	Member of the Institute of Pure Chiropractic
MIPTI	Member of the Independent Professional Therapists International
MIRMT	Member of the Independent Register of Manipulative Therapists
MIROM	Member of the International Register of Oriental Medicine
MISPH	Member of the International Society for Professional Hypnosis
MISPT	Member of the International Society of Polarity Therapists
MLCOM	Member of the College of Osteopathic Medicine (doctors only)
MNAHP	Member of the National Association of Hypnotists & Psychotherapists
MNCP	Member of the National Council of Psychotherapists & Hypnotherapy
MNIMH	Member of the National Institute of Medical Herbalists
MNTOS	Member of the Natural Therapeutic Osteopathic Society
MPEPA	Member of the Polarity Energetics Practitioners Association
MPNLP	NLP Master Practitioner
MRad A	Member of the Radionics Association
MRCHM	Member of the Register of Chinese Herbal Medicine
MRCN	Member of the Register of Clinical Nutritionists
MRCP	Member of the Royal College of Physicians
MRCS	Member of the Royal College of Surgeons
MRH	Member of the Register of Herbalists

MRN	Member of the General Council & Register of Naturopaths
MRO	Member of the Register of Osteopaths
MRSH	Member of the Royal Society of Health
MRSS	Member of the Register of the Shiatsu Society
MRTA	Member of the Relaxation Therapy Association
MRTCM	Member of the Register of Traditional Chinese Medicine
MSAAc	Member of the Society of Auricular Acupuncturists
MSAPP	Member of the Society of Advanced Psychotherapy Practitioners
MSBM	Member of the Society of Biophysical Medicine
MSF	Member of the Smae Institute (Swedish massage & chiropody)
MSHP	Member of the Society of Holistic Practitioners
MSS	Member of the Shiatsu Society
MSTAT	Member of the Society of Teachers of the Alexander Technique
MTAcs	Member of the Traditional Acupuncture Society
MWFH	Member of the World Federation of Hypnotherapists
ND	Diploma in Naturopathy
NFSH	National Federation of Spiritual Healers
NRHP	National Register of Hypnotherapists & Psychotherapists
PGCE	Post Graduate Certificate of Education
RGN	Registered General Nurse
RIr	Registered Iridologist
RMANM	Registered Member of the Association of Natural Medicines
RMAPC	Registered Member of the Association of Psychic Counsellors
RMN	Registered Mental Nurse

RPT	Registered Polarity Therapist
RSHom	Registered with the Society of Homoeopaths
RTCM	Register of Traditional Chinese Medicine
SAPP	Society of Advanced Psychotherapy Practitioners
SCM	State Certified Midwife
SPAG	Shirley Price Aromatherapy GP
SRCL	State Registered Chiropodist
SRN	State Registered Nurse
SRP	State Registered Physiotherapist
STAT	Society of Teachers of the Alexander Technique
TAS	Traditional Acupuncture Society
TDHA	Tisserand Diploma in Holistic Aromatherapy
WFH	World Federation of Healers

INDEX